BORN WITH ONE FOOT IN THE GRAVE

HARRY AND CINDY GREINER

This book is dedicated to the Greiner's that have gone before that they may never be forgotten and to the ones in the present that bring hope for the future.

JOE'S FATHERS DAY CARD 2001

DAD

I WANT TO THANK YOU FOR ALWAYS
BEING THERE FOR ME. EVEN WHEN I
DIDN'T APPRECIATE IT. THE WHOLE
YOU GETTING SICK THING MADE ME
REALIZE NOT ONLY HOW I WASN'T GOOD
TO YOU, BUT HOW MUCH YOU AND I ARE
ALIKE. SO WHEN YOU WERE SICK, I
FELT LIKE I WAS WATCHING MYSELF BE
SICK AND THAT'S WHY I COULDN'T
HANDLE BEING AROUND IT. I JUST
WANT YOU TO KNOW HOW MUCH I LOVE
YOU. I'M GLAD I CAN COME TO YOU
ABOUT STUFF IN LIFE NOW WHERE I
GUESS I WAS AFRAID TO BEFORE. SO
THANKS FOR EVERYTHING AND HAPPY
FARTHER'S DAY!

HARRY

My life began much like a scene out of the old TV show "The Andy Griffith Show." A small southern Ohio town with a mechanic you could trust to keep you safe on the road. An insurance man who really cared about you and your family and looked out for your interests to keep you safe from the unfortunate things that can happen in life. A doctor who knew your family, and did his best to take care of you and your loved ones in times of illness or injury. Neighbors who were there for you when you needed them. Who always said "Good morning" to you and took the time to talk with you. Now money and getting ahead is the most important thing to everyone. Even using it to kill, injure, and to maim people.

FORTY YEARS LATER. . .

I'm lying in my bed listening to the faint sound of a lonesome train whistle in the distance. My thoughts are "do I want to live or die?" My past was a nightmare, my present was even worse. Did I have any future? And if so, by some sort of miracle, what would that be like? I thought, "it's so easy to take your own life, and yet so hard." Dear God, what has brought me to this horrible reality? To have to make such a horrible decision on my own. I love my family so much, and I never meant to bring this nightmare into their lives..

CHAPTER ONE

I met Harry in the summer of 1973. We worked together in the office at a folding box company in Sandusky, Ohio. He was a packaging designer and I worked in accounting. His art teacher at Ehove Joint Vocational School had referred him there. I had been working there about a year when Harry started to work there. I guess you could say that I can thank the old TV series "Dark Shadows" for drawing my attention to him, because to me he looked just like a character on that show called "Quentin Collins".

The first week Harry worked with me; a reporter from the newspaper came and did an article on him about his new life after

3

having a kidney transplant. I had no clue what that was at the time. When Harry explained it to me, I was scared; it seemed like something out of a science fiction movie, and I didn't understand it.

Harry would later tell me that the first time he saw me walk down the hall; he knew he wanted to marry me. As soon as we met, we started dating and fell instantly in love with each other, and were engaged to be married within half a year.

I had gone to meet his family shortly after we first started dating. Harry's mom was named Hilda; she had come from Germany with his dad after World War II. Her speech was a comical mix of southern drawl with a German accent. He had six sisters, five still at home, and his Dad, Bob, had died in 1956 of kidney disease when he had been only twenty-eight years old.

Hilda decided that she was going to tell me the very heart-

4

breaking tale of the Greiner's and she told me every gory detail. I have never known to this day why she told me this story almost the first time she met me. Had she wanted to scare me away or did she want to know if I had the guts to deal with it? I never asked her, and now it will forever remain a mystery.

The Greiner's had lived on Howard Hill Road in Ripley, Ohio since the 1840's. The original Greiner's had come from Germany to live in Ohio because the hills there reminded them of home. You could see the farmhouse they lived in sitting just over the ridge of a very high hill. It was a two story white house with a tin roof and fancy trim on the front porch. It still stands today, being only slightly remodeled on the outside.

A single lane road ran upward at such a sharp incline that it was impassable in the winter. A smaller house sat off to the side of the main house. A long road ran beside a cluster of barn buildings that led back to the 180 acres of farmland that they owned. They had always been a close-knit family and built their house to be a thing of beauty.

Harry's grandfather Oscar was the youngest child born in the third generation of Greiner's to live in that house. In 1921, he married Ollie Belle Bryan and brought her to live at the house with his mother and father. They had four children, Elbert, Lester, Herman, and Robert, who would become Harry's father. Never did he imagine that his house and his life would one day be so full of tragedy.

In 1931, Ollie Belle died of kidney disease at the age of twenty-eight, and Oscar bought ten plots in Maplewood Cemetery in Ripley so that even in death his family would be together. Little did he know then how soon his family would join their mother there. Oscar was desolate and was left to raise his sons alone.

The years went by, his mother and father both died, and his sons were growing up. When our country entered World War II, Elbert was drafted. When the troop train pulled out of Ripley, he looked out the window, and had a very strong feeling of dread and said he knew that he would never see home again. In 1945, he was killed in France by a land mine. His body was brought home to be buried in the family plot.

In February of 1946, Bob joined the army and was sent to Germany to be part of the forces over there during the occupation after World War II. In December of that year, Bob received word that his brother Herman had died at home of kidney disease. Herman was only twenty-three years old and he and his wife Nancy had been married for only a year and a half. This was a terrible blow; he could not even come home for the funeral.

In 1947, Bob met Hilda Schmid in Germany. Hilda was born there in Augsburg, and was a short petite woman with dark brown hair. They fell in love and were married in 1948 in the Catholic Church in Germany and again by the United States army as was the custom in those days in order for Hilda to be able to come to the United States and live.

Bob arrived in the United States with the army in 1948 and was discharged. Hilda came later by plane and arrived in New York. She was ready to start a whole new life after being raised in war torn Germany. She was soon to be very disappointed. Germans at that time thought the American people were very rich.

Bob, his brother Les and his wife Mary drove to New York to meet Hilda's plane and somehow they missed each other. Although Hilda spoke very little English, she found a way to call Oscar and to get to Ripley, Ohio from New

York. She was taken by taxi to a farmhouse on the top of Howard's Hill Road. The place looked dark and deserted. Oscar came outside with a lantern to meet her. It was then she realized that there was no electricity and no indoor plumbing. She wondered what she had gotten herself into.

Oscar and his two sons and their wives lived together on the farm as the family had for generations. Everything belonged to Oscar now. The Greiner's were primarily tobacco farmers as that has always been the main crop grown in Ripley. They are famous for their tobacco warehouses.

The women cooked, cleaned, and worked the fields with the men. Hilda despised it there, but had a friend in Nancy, Herman's widow. They had to wash their clothes in a big iron pot over a fire in the yard or on a scrub board. The water in the kitchen came from a hand pump that they cranked. The milk was kept cold by putting it in a bucket that was hanging in the well.

It took Hilda awhile to adjust to American ways, and find the things she needed to buy. Things in America were named differently than in Germany. She had never even seen a rocking chair and was scared to death when she first sat in it because she thought it was broken.

Hilda and Bob lived on the farm until after their first child Carol was born in 1950. It was always a joke that Carol had been delivered by a vet. The doctor raised horses, so Hilda thought he was a vet. It was years later that we found out that he really was a doctor. Hilda tended to mix things up that way.

Harry was born when the family lived on North Pole Road. He was the only one of their kids to be born in the hospital. They lived too far away from a doctor so he was born in Maysville, Kentucky, which had the nearest hospital.

Hilda named her only son Harry after the doctor because she said that Bob didn't come in time to help her pick a name for the birth certificate. Harry's middle name is Clarence, the same as his grandfather's. Carol could not say the name Harry, and thought his head looked like a pumpkin. So from then on, his nickname was Punk and it has stuck to this day.

Hilda and Bob then decided to move into town to a house at 202 N. Second Street. It hadn't been lived in for years. It was a spooky old run down place, with an overgrown backyard that looked like a forest. They worked hard to clear it out and clean up the inside.

In 1954, they had twin girls, Norma Jean and Nancy Jane named after his brother Herman's wife Nancy Stivers. The twins were born premature as they sometimes are and Norma had to be kept near the stove to keep her warm, since she was the smallest. With Hilda's mixed up stories, it has always been a joke that Norma had come baked in an oven.

In 1955, Bob started feeling sick. When he went to the doctor, he was told he had kidney disease like his brother. At the time, it was called Bright's disease or glomerulonephritis. There was no cure for it and the only way to prolong your life was to maintain a certain diet and rest. Hilda and Bob were sick with grief. They were both very young with four children under the age of six to raise. Bob knew what was coming and refused to follow the diet or rest. He said he was a dead man anyway.

In the fall of 1956, he became so ill he was sent to the veteran's hospital in Cincinnati. Harry's Uncle Les, who was by that time divorced, took Hilda back and forth to the hospital to sit with Bob. The kids would play outside while Hilda visited their Dad.

Hilda questioned how Bob could have gotten into the army with this disease since it shows up in your urine years before you become sick with it. The Veterans Administration said he didn't have it at the time and the two years he spent in the army did not harm him in any way. They said he would have died anyway. Back then you had to take their word for it. With what I now know about this disease, it was a lie and a cover up. It would have shown up in the urine sample during the army physical.

The doctors told Hilda that they had a brand new treatment at the hospital called a dialysis machine. If Bob's heart could take it, he might be able to live longer. This machine could filter the poisons out of his blood. He would have to be able to be on the machine for two hours in order for it to work. The machine was in the hospital basement and took up an entire room.

Hilda and Les waited outside in the hall during the treatment. An hour and a half later, they heard a commotion. They were yanking tubes out of Bob and blood was flying all over the walls and over everyone in the room. They rushed Bob through tunnels to the other side of the hospital. They made Hilda wait while they drained the rest of his blood out of the tubes and made her carry bottles of his blood to the room where they took her husband. This is something they would do in a horror movie, and it would haunt Hilda for the rest of her life.

After that, all kinds of specialists came to see Bob and said he was just too far gone to help. Hilda begged them to put him back on the machine, but they said his blood pressure was just too high, and it would kill him.

In 1956, this was a horrible way to die. The poisons consumed his body until he was delirious. He hemorrhaged out of his eyes from the high blood pressure. They strapped him in his bed with metal cuffs and he fought so hard there was no skin left on his wrists. At the time, I was horrified to imagine watching someone you love die that horrible way. I can now unfortunately envision it.

On November 15, 1956, Hilda and Les were called to the hospital; Bob was dying. They rushed there and Les waited outside, as he could not stand to watch another brother die. Bob sat up in bed suddenly, and seemed completely normal. He tried to tell Hilda he was sorry, and died.

Les and Hilda went back to her house that night and they were heartbroken. They were sitting in the living room, when all of a sudden the lamps went out one at a time until three lights went out. Then they all came back on in exactly the same order. It was a very strange thing to happen and it scared them, since Bob was the third brother to die.

The last memory Harry has of his father is of him lying in bed sick and sitting on the bed next to him playing. And he remembers his Dad's funeral. Hilda took the kids to the funeral and they had nightmares for years afterward. He was buried in the family plot with his mother and brothers. The Greiner's had so much tragedy in their lives, and these were the shadows that haunted Harry's early years.

Shortly after that, Harry's grandfather came to live with them. There was no one left willing to do the farming and Oscar was getting older. He sold the land and the property on Howard Hill Road, and I'm sure he felt he let his ancestors down.

He was good to his grandkids, but very sad and heartbroken about losing all of his family. There is a picture of him with Carol, Harry, Nancy and Norma, and he looks so sad and defeated. I am sure he probably thought his grandchildren would have kidney disease and die also. The man lived the life of Job in the bible. Everything was taken from him, his wife, his three sons and his land.

Hilda didn't have much money after that. They grew a big garden in the backyard and ate mostly vegetables and potatoes. They even paid their doctor bills with vegetables. On Sunday, they usually had a big meal of fried chicken. Oscar would go hunting and bring home squirrel or rabbit to eat. Harry had a lot of fun as a kid growing up in a small town. He never realized then that his life would hold so much pain and sickness.

When Harry was eight years old, he had scarlatina and the house was quarantined. All the bedding had to be burned once he was well. In those days, they put a sign on the door when someone had a communicable disease. When he was ten, his appendix burst and he had to go to the hospital to have them removed. Hilda once told me that everything with Harry was an emergency, even when he was a child. I think when you have surgery as a child you learn to dread going to the hospital.

Hilda did the best she could to keep food on the table, in spite of everything. They all had good friends in Ripley. Hilda was best friends with her neighbor Phyllis Myers; they spent a lot of time together because Phyllis' husband had a job that took him all over the country. Carol would bring friends over, and Hilda would dance with them to the songs on "American Bandstand" on Saturday afternoons. Hilda was a good dancer and would teach the girls some German dances.

Harry had a good friend from school, David Gast, and hung around with Phyllis' sons from across the street. Nancy and Norma were identical in every way. They were shy and played with some girls down the street.

When Harry was twelve, Hilda was working in a bakery. It was there that she met John Ruggles and she brought him home to meet the kids. A short time later, they decided to get married. It was fun for them to have John around at first. They now had a car and could go places. John used to take Harry with him on his bakery route.

Since Hilda was going to be remarried, she asked Les to come and take his Dad home to live with him. Les had also gotten married again, and he came and picked up his Dad. It would be years before Harry saw Les again, and it would be a crisis that would bring them back together.

So now, thirty-eight years later I ask myself why anyone would tell this story to someone who loved their son. Why did she want to drive me away with this heinous story? Well, the story of his Dad's death scared me to death all right. Nothing was ever the same again. I was haunted by it. I loved Harry and was torn apart thinking about our future and the children we would have.

Hilda showed me pictures of the Greiner's that had died. There was one of Nancy and Herman. I could see how much Nancy loved him and for some odd reason I felt an instant connection to her. Not to Hilda, but to someone I did not even know. I thought I would end up like Nancy, with a husband that would die young.

That is all I got out of the story. I didn't understand what a kidney transplant was really, or that it had saved his life. I just thought that at some point it would not work and he would die.

Hilda told the story in such a matter of fact manner that it seemed like she didn't even care. I would realize later that denial was her defense against the horror she had been through twice with kidney disease. She had also just lost her second husband, John Ruggles, the year before. He had died of a blockage to the heart after having dental surgery.

Hilda had their three small children to raise alone again. JoAnn was eight, Kelley was three, and Chris was two years old. Nancy, Norma, and Harry were still at home and Carol had been married and moved out a couple of years before. Hilda had lost both husbands before she was even married ten years.

Instead of giving Harry John's car when he died, Hilda made him buy it from her. It was a green 1967 LTD and not in the best of shape. He had to learn about car repair in a hurry. And since Harry had the only car and Hilda couldn't drive, she always wanted Harry to stay at home because she was afraid that something would happen to the kids and she wouldn't be able to get to the hospital. Harry and I could not understand this paranoia at the time. We just wanted to have a life. However, I now understand that Hilda was afraid to be alone because so much had happened to her.

Hilda's house was a depressing place at the time. It was always full of doom and gloom. All the rooms in the house had this dark paneling on the walls and Hilda would sit in the house all day with the curtains closed to the world. She was very depressed.

Six months after Harry and I started going together, we were engaged and went to look at wedding rings together. I was still upset about Harry's medical background. It sadly clouded all my thoughts at that time. It was supposed to be a happy time, but it wasn't. But I was in love with him and knew I couldn't live without him. It was as if destiny was calling and I was being swept along with it.

Hilda had a lot more stories

to tell. When Harry was thirteen, he broke out in a rash and a urine test showed albium or protein in his urine, which is a sign that your kidneys aren't functioning the way they should be. Hilda was so scared. The doctor had told her at the time Bob died that the disease was not hereditary.

Harry was taken to the hospital in Cincinnati. They did extensive allergy tests and a kidney biopsy. He was scared and fought the anesthesia. So he was awake during the whole procedure. It was very painful having a needle stuck in your back. And in those days, they used a much larger needle for a biopsy than they do today. Harry didn't understand what was going on. He was there for two weeks.

After that, his life changed overnight. He was allergic to everything imaginable, most likely because his kidney' were failing. He didn't know it, but the doctor had told his Mom and John that he also had kidney disease and would not live past the age of twenty-one. The only hope he had was a new operation that was done only in the bigger city hospitals. It was a kidney transplant, and it was only done on twins at the time.

They advised them not to tell Harry because he would not be able to take this kind of news. Hilda knew she had to protect him and watch him carefully to keep him alive as long as she could. She had seen this before, and she was devastated.

After that, Harry was coddled and he hated it. He saw no sense in the way he was being treated. His new bike was taken away, he wasn't allowed out in the cold, or to do anything he had enjoyed before. He started high school the next year in Ripley, but could only go half days.

During that first year in high school, he was told the family was moving to Norwalk,

24

Ohio. He didn't want to leave his friends or his hometown. They were moving to be near a large hospital that could help him. but Harry still didn't know anything was wrong with him. In the fall of 1965, it seemed they just up and and moved overnight.

Harry was not permitted to go to school at all then, which was just as well because he hated explaining to the other kids why he didn't go to school all day; he didn't know the answer to that anyway. They decided that he should be taught at home for two years. The doctors thought school would be too much of a physical strain for him. The thinking was so different back then.

Harry became really shy and didn't have any friends except the ones Carol brought over. Harry had a big crush on Carol's friend Rosemary, whose brother had died of the same kidney disease, nephritis. He went to the prom with her and it was the highlight of his life at the time. He realized later that she probably felt sorry for him because he was going to die. Carol was the only one of his sisters who knew he was sick. Hilda wanted Carol to keep an eye on him.

Life at home with John was not ideal either. He was not his real Dad, and Harry and his sisters tended to take their mother's side when she and John had an argument. There were a lot of problems, and John started to drink. The police were at their house a lot for domestic disputes.

Carol, Nancy, Norma, and Harry were locked in their rooms a lot, and were not allowed to make any noise. Their meals were brought to their bedroom doors. Carol would just climb out the window and sneak away to be with her friends. But she got a beating when she came back.

John always took his daughter JoAnn's side, no matter what she said, and Harry was usually the one that got the beating because of her. Until the day Harry got old enough to back John up against the wall and told him to keep his hands off him. That was the end of the abuse.

During that time the doctors suggested Harry go to a Bureau of Vocational Rehabilitation facility in Cincinnati. He could hear his mother and the social worker talking about him and his Dad, but couldn't quite catch what they were saying. They thought that if he possibly survived, he would be disabled and need an occupation.

So one night they packed his suitcase and John took him to Cincinnati to the BVR facility. They told Harry that he had to go because of his allergies. There were a lot of older people with handicaps. They all slept in a room with many beds like a dormitory. During the day they went to workshops to be evaluated for a type of work that they had a talent for and would be able to do with their particular type of handicap.

He was sixteen years old and in a place where people had no arms and legs. He was scared, confused, and wanted to go home. He did not belong there with those people, because as far as he knew, there was nothing much wrong with him. It seemed backward and old fashioned. This particular memory of his always makes me cry. He didn't know why he had been put in that place. But Hilda and John did what they thought was best for him at the time.

He was there for a month. John came to pick him up and on the way home they went through Ripley, and stopped to see a few friends. Harry said it was really strange being there and his childhood seemed like a dream. No one was even on the streets and it looked like a ghost town. Things were always so old fashioned there anyway. Everything seemed so different, but then he thought that maybe it was he who had changed, not the town. His life had changed drastically and he had been through so many things since the day he had left there.

After he came home, he was so glad to see his family again. Later that night he was sitting in his room. It was a minute after midnight. He happened to turn his head toward the window, which started at the floor and went all the way up to the ceiling. He saw a figure float in with deep-seated evil eyes. It's eyes seemed to embed themselves into Harry's eyes and his mind. And in those eyes, he could see a whole other world. He could not move or say a word.

He could hear Nancy and Norma in the other room and couldn't call out to them. Then it just floated out the same way it came in. Harry thought hours had gone by, but only a few minutes had passed. He now wonders if it could have been a harbinger of impending death.

Harry waited for the results from the BVR. They said he was good at drafting and art, so it was decided he could go back to school for his Junior and Senior year. They enrolled him in Ehove Vocational School in Avery, Ohio. He wanted to take drafting but the class was full, so he decided to take commercial art.

He felt like a normal person for the first time in years. He had friends and could go to school, but he was still told he could not do a lot of thing. He was not allowed to go to the football games because it was too damp outside and he might get sick. There really wasn't much he could do about it, but he resented it. His friends were told that he was sick so they would understand what was going on with him. But Harry was mad and getting suspicious. He was not even allowed to get his driver's license until he was 18.

And Harry himself was feeling

sick by now. He was so tired all the time. He barely got home from school before he passed out on his bed changing his clothes. He was losing his appetite and his allergies were so bad he could hardly breathe at all, even with the allergy shots. He constantly used nasal spray and even that didn't work anymore.

He kept asking his Mom what his Dad had died of, but Hilda would always change the subject. Finally, one day she wrote it on a piece of paper, but grabbed it away so fast that he didn't quite catch the spelling. He went to the library to look it up and figured out that it was kidney disease. He hoped he didn't have the same thing and it worried him.

In 1971, Harry graduated from high school, only a year later than he originally should have. After that, he started looking for a job. Carol got him a job as an orderly at the local hospital. He really didn't like hospitals. He had been in one when his appendix had burst when he was in the fifth grade and then when he had the kidney biopsy. He never wanted to be in a hospital again.

He saw all kinds of sick and dying people, and it was very upsetting. It might not have been so bad if he didn't feel as sick as the patients did. He had to quit because he felt so weak and nauseous, but he never told Hilda and John the real reason.

One day shortly after he was home awhile, Harry and Hilda were watching a television show about a girl who was going to die. She asked Harry if he would want to know if he was dying. He said he wouldn't want to know and didn't know why she was asking. Then she started telling him that there were graves in Ripley that his grandfather had bought and still belonged to them. He didn't pay much attention to her at the time.

CHAPTER TWO

A couple months after that Harry was getting really sick. He would be driving and everything on the road would swirl in front of his eyes. It was the result of high blood pressure and the poisons in his blood building up because his kidneys were failing, but he thought he had an ulcer. He had no appetite and had lost weight. He never told anyone how sick he really was because he didn't want to go to the hospital.

I'm sure his mother noticed. At the time that she told me this story; I wondered why she didn't do anything. I thought she should have taken him to the doctor, because she knew he was sick. Now years later, I understand, she was afraid and in denial. I would do the same thing years later with my own son.

Finally, he had to go to the doctor because he was so sick. When he came out of the office, Hilda went in to talk to the doctor in private and came out sobbing. She knew the end was coming. There are no words to express what she must have been feeling. She told Harry he had to be admitted to the hospital, and to her he was going there to die, just like his Dad had.

Harry told her not to cry, after all he only had an ulcer, which only made her cry all the harder. He felt so bad by now, he didn't even care where they took him, he just wanted to be well.

In the hospital, Harry threw up four or five times every hour. He drank barium for x-rays, and had a million tests. And he was very, very sick. He became so upset, they tried to give him shots to calm him down, but it had the opposite effect.

Everyone's voices sounded like chickens in fast motion, and he felt like he was losing his mind. He couldn't talk to tell anyone what was wrong with him, and finally they realized that instead of making him calm the medicine was making him feel frantic. It was a horrible and scary time for him, not knowing why he was so sick.

Everyone came to see him, Carol and her husband Mike, and all his friends, Jackson and Gary and Terry. They hardly recognized him he looked so bad. Harry was in the hospital for a couple of weeks. He turned twenty on September 3, 1971 and spent his birthday in the hospital. He thought he could never feel any worse, but that was nothing compared to what the days ahead would bring.

Then he was sent to the Cleveland Clinic, the only place close at the time that did kidney transplants. He could barely walk, and he was so nauseous. John and Hilda took him there in the car. He knew by now that he didn't have an ulcer, but he still didn't know what was wrong with him.

They took him into the emergency room, and the nurse there said they must have the wrong chart. It couldn't possibly be Harry, because the man's vitals on the chart belonged to a dead man. They took him into an exam room, and it took forever for a doctor to come in and look at him.

The doctor kept asking Harry why was he there, what was wrong with him and what medicines did he take. He just shook his head and sighed because he had no answers to any of those questions. John and Hilda came in and explained, but Harry couldn't hear the answers. They took tests for a few hours and Harry went back out in the waiting room to sit with John and Hilda. There were so many sick people there moaning and groaning. He tried to keep his mind off of them.

They finally decided to admit him, but when they found out he didn't have any health insurance, they refused to let him in the hospital. John yelled at them and asked them what kind of a place this was that puts dying people out on the street. After a lot of argument, John threatened to expose them to the news media. The clinic then decided they would let him be admitted.

Harry hadn't eaten in a couple of weeks now and still couldn't keep anything down. After awhile, he just didn't eat because he thought, what's the use; it will only come back up anyway. There was nothing left to throw up except the bile in the lining of his stomach.

One of the nurses on the floor would come in all the time and tease him about having a girlfriend. She would say, "Are you a virgin, boy?" He was so sick he never answered her, so she tried to touch him in an inappropriate way. Finally, someone passed by in the hall, so she stopped. This same nurse started getting mad at him for throwing up so much. She told him he was going to change his bed himself if he threw up one more time. The next time he threw up, she threw the puke bucket under his bed.

When Hilda and John came back in the room and heard of these incidents, they immediately complained to the hospital staff about this nurse. They were told she was fired. Thirty-five years later, we would see this nurse sitting in the hospital cafeteria. She told us she had been promoted back then to surgical nurse.

So, apparently when there is a complaint about misconduct at the Cleveland Clinic, they hide the employee until the situation blows over and then promote them to a higher position. What does that say about the clinic's standard of care? Not a whole lot.

They had to measure his urine, and save some for the tests they did on him. They also kept track of how much he drank. By now he had the dry heaves, and he could not sleep at night because he was so sick. Doctors in groups and of all nationalities would come in, talk in another language, and just shake their heads. They scared Harry to death, a practice they have always excelled at.

Finally, someone told him he had the same disease as his Dad; they assumed he already knew. Harry knew then he was going to die. Twenty years old, and he never even had a chance to have a life. They told him he could have a kidney transplant; it was his only chance, but he didn't believe them. His own parents had lied to him and he thought they were too. It was the most terrifying moment of his life, but it explained a lot of things about the unusual way he had grown up. He had been cheated out of his past and he had no future.

They moved Harry to the floor with the kidney patients. He was in a private room with only a brick wall for a view outside the window. There were no days and nights, just endless hours of sickness. He was urinating less and less. His kidneys were decaying quickly. With this disease, the glomerulus in the kidneys scar up and die off. These are the very delicate blood filtering parts of your kidneys.

He couldn't eat, couldn't stand up because he was so weak, and was losing weight fast. There were no IV's for dehydration because his kidneys would not filter out any fluid. His whole body itched from the poisons that weren't filtering out of his body. With the vomiting, itching, and nausea, he was getting hysterical and started to wish for death.

Finally, after a month, the doctors prescribed a pill to calm his stomach and stop the vomiting. Why would they let someone in that condition just lie there so sick and simply ignore him for a month? It just seemed like torture to me.

Of course, the pills had side effects. Harry fainted outside in the hall and was brought back to bed. His words were very slurred, and they thought he had a lump on the back of his head. He couldn't tell them it was always there. He was afraid they would be cutting into the back of his head next. They finally realized that the pills were doing this to him.

Harry could not stand to be left alone. He pressed his buzzer for the nurse all night long. Either Hilda or John stayed with him, which was difficult for both of them. John had a job to go to and Hilda had five kids at home to take care of. Chris was only nine months old at the time. John missed a lot of days of work, but for the first time in a long time he was very good to Harry, and he appreciated it.

Hilda was reliving a terrible nightmare. She would stay at the hospital for days with no clean clothes and very little to eat. When you have no money to spend, you might as well be in the desert at the clinic. The food, parking and hotels in the clinic are very expensive.

The doctors finally decided to put Harry on dialysis. He had to be on peritoneal at first, and in those days it was a heinous procedure. A tube was inserted into your abdomen until it was in your peritoneal cavity. They knew it was in the right place when you felt a cramp in your rectum.

Attached to the tube was a five-gallon glass bottle of peritoneal dialysis fluid hung on a stand. Cleansing fluid called dialysate was put into your peritoneal cavity with a pump. This pulled the waste and extra fluids out of the patient's blood into the peritoneal cavity. The fluid would remain in there for a certain amount of time called dwell time. Then another tube drew the fluid and the poisons back out and into another bottle. This process was controlled with timers and clamps. Then they stuck a plastic stopper in your stomach to keep the hole open for the next dialysis treatment. That button drove Harry nuts, it was so uncomfortable.

During this time Hilda and John brought Harry's sisters to see him. He was so glad to see everyone that he couldn't stop crying. He visited with them awhile and then he kissed them goodbye, knowing he might never see them again. He went back to his room and thought about being home again. He had been sick for so long, he had almost forgotten what it was like to be at home and feel well.

It wasn't long before he had to go on dialysis again. The button had been taken out of his stomach because he couldn't stand it. Now a new hole had to be made. A new technician was there that day. He tried repeatedly to get the tube in the right hole. They finally inserted it, and filled him up with fluid, but it wouldn't come back out.

Instead of correcting their mistake, they just took him back to his room. He was so bloated with dialysis fluid by the next morning; they had to take him back downstairs to drain it out. Harry said, "I'm not going. I just wish I could die, I've had enough."

Hilda made him go, and told the doctors what he had said. Then a psychiatrist came to see him, and asked him all kinds of questions. "Do you hate your life? Do you hate your father for giving you this disease?" He didn't understand why he was being asked all those questions, and they just went on and on.

Back in the 1970's, kidney transplants were still new.

Hospital care should have been excellent, but is was more like the early days of the century at the clinic. The really horrible thing is that things should have improved by the year 2006, but as we saw firsthand, the patients are still experimented on at the Cleveland Clinic. If anything is going to save you there, it will be the hand of God, not their good care.

Harry laid there in bed at the time thinking about what some of the other dialysis patients had told him. Some of them came in several times a week, had a job, lived at home and had a semi normal life. And they did this for years. This didn't seem like any life to Harry even though it was the only way for now to stay alive. He had never been able to have a normal life, and that didn't seem like one either.

A Chinese doctor came in one day and told him about another type of dialysis called hemodialysis. It would require having what they then called a shunt put in your arm. An artery is cut in the arm and two Teflon tipped tubes are inserted into an artery and vein and joined on the outside with a straight connector. The two tubes are then connected to a dialysis machine.

The blood flows out of your arm into the machine where it is cleaned out with filters and chemicals. It then flows back in through the other tube into your arm cleaned and free of poisons. There was a high risk back then of the tubes being disconnected and you had to carry stainless steel shunt clips around with you to clamp the arteries so you would not bleed to death. Fistulas were not used until after 1976.

Harry really wanted to be on this type of dialysis. He knew it would be less painful, but you had to be on a list because there was a limited amount of machines. They should have put a shunt in his arm in advance, but as always, they are disorganized and never think of the patient or their comfort first.

So when the day came for him to be on this type of dialysis he was taken downstairs and suddenly realized how they were going to put him on the machine. There was a large tube lying next to the machine, and Harry started to sweat. They numbed his groin, and shoved a tube in there up to his femoral artery. It was an uncomfortable feeling and he was still itching from the poisons in his bloodstream and wanted so badly to scratch, but he couldn't move at all. This procedure went on for six hours, three times a week for several weeks. He started to feel slightly better after the first treatment and was able to sleep for the first time in months.

Finally, the day came when a shunt was put in his arm. Since Harry never fell asleep during any procedure he ever had, he told them to just numb his arm. By the time they cut the artery and blood was squirting everywhere, he felt like passing out. But he endured the pain with the thought that this was better than a tube shoved up your groin. How sad to be happy for the worst of two evils. It was soon over and dialysis was a breeze compared to the other methods.

The next operation would be a nephrectomy, the removal of his diseased kidneys. He thought it would never end, tubes and needles and knives. The clinic told him to go home for a few weeks to regain his strength before the next operation. His morale was really low.

John picked him up at the hospital. All the leaves had turned their fall colors. His attitude began to change a little. He knew he wasn't going to die now, and only the future held any promise. Harry has had this attitude in all the years I have known him. He is always striving for something better in life.

Harry went into the house and hugged everybody. He was home, a place he thought he would never see again. Hilda had made a bed down-stairs for him so he could watch TV. He still didn't have much of an appetite, but it was much better than before he went into the hospital.

A dialysis diet is tough, no salt, potassium, and not much protein. The fluid restriction was the worst; he could only have a couple of small cups of water a day. So now he was home and he thought he wouldn't be so sick anymore, but he still wasn't well. He could eat breakfast, but lunch and supper were bad; he would be sick and nervous especially when he had to go on dialysis that night. The treatments started at ten at night and lasted until four or five in the morning.

He was still going to

Cleveland three times a week for dialysis. He would be sick afterwards for a day, and by the time he felt better it was time to go back again. John had spent a lot of time driving back and forth the sixty miles to Cleveland, so some of their friends offered to take Harry back and forth to dialysis so John could go back to work.

Since Harry had no insurance, the cost of all his medical bills and dialysis treatments were piling up. The newspapers were doing articles on Harry and his family. The civic groups were doing fundraisers, and the local doctor set up a bank account called the "Legacy for Life" for Harry and other families in critical medical situations. This fund still exists today. A lot of people donated money to this fund, food for the family and nine people offered to be kidney donors. To this day Harry still doesn't know their names. This is our opportunity to thank them for their kindness and unselfishness. He received hundreds of cards with money in it to help his family. The people of Norwalk were really kind and generous.

When Harry was still in the hospital, Hilda and John started looking for Harry's Uncle Les. They knew he needed a kidney transplant and a family member was the best choice. They called every person they knew in Ripley to find him, but were told he had moved to a nearby town. They called the utility companies, and the state highway patrol to help find him. Les was living in Seaman, Ohio at the time.

As soon as they found him, he agreed right away to be tested to be a kidney donor. He was the only one left of his brothers, and he would have done anything to help his brother Bob's son. At the time, Les didn't know for sure if his own children would have this disease, but his wife's side of the family had a lot of relatives, and he was all Harry had.

Hilda and Carol had both volunteered to be donors, but they didn't match, and Nancy and Norma were too young. Thank God they were, because of what would happen later. It was and still is a blessing to have a live donor. The number of people needing transplants far outweighed the number of kidneys available. That number has tripled in the last forty years. There are now approximately 114,000 people waiting for a kidney transplant.

The donor had to undergo many tests. Their kidneys had to be healthy and free of disease. In those days the donor was considered an A, B, or C match. An A being an identical twin, a B was a mother or father, and a C was a close relative. Les was a C match and his blood type O, the same as Harry's. This was called tissue typing. One of the tests was an angiogram, which involved pushing a tube into your groin, up through an artery to the kidney. Then they shot an ultra-violet light through the tube to see the kidney. It was painful, and it burned.

Les was told the risks of having one kidney. You can live perfectly well that way, but you have to take care of yourself. I believe he would have done this for Harry no matter what. This was the last thing he could do to help his brothers. Les had helped raise Harry's Dad, who had been only three years old when their mother had died at age twenty-eight. The last time Harry had seen Les was when he had came to take his father home to live with him. Harry's grandfather had died at age seventy-two.

Back then you could eat any-thing you wanted while you were on the machine, the theory being it was being filtered back out again any- way. He was too sick to eat, and could only keep from throwing up until the last half hour.

Dialysis was hard on him. The

shunt in his arm would get really warm when blood ran through it. His blood pressure would drop so low, he had to be taken to the car in a wheelchair. He would just go home and collapse into bed.

Even though he was nauseous, he would fall asleep. But he wanted to live, and if this was the way, so be it. He knew that he had to do everything he was told if he wanted to have a successful transplant.

Friends came to visit to cheer him up. When he was still in the hospital, his best friend from Ripley, David Gast and his wife Barb came to visit him. They had been friends since they went to grade school together at the Catholic school in Ripley. It meant a lot to Harry.

Just before Thanksgiving in 1971, it was time for Harry to go back into the hospital for his nephrectomy, the removal of his diseased kidneys. It was scheduled for November 23, at 9:30 a.m. He was so nervous the night before his hands were shaking. When the operation was over, he was in intensive care for awhile. He spent Thanksgiving in the hospital. No turkey, but his Mom and John came to visit. After about a week, he went home.

A short time afterwards, he developed a fever. He had an incision down the front of his chest and stomach and it had infection oozing out. The doctor opened a two-inch section of it up in the exam room and showed them how to take care of it. Hilda had to pour peroxide in the incision and pack it with gauze. I swear you cannot have anything done at the Cleveland Clinic without getting an infection.

Les had been accepted to be Harry's kidney donor, and he felt very blessed to not have to be on a transplant list. The transplant surgery was to be done on December 16, 1971. Because of the infection, the transplant had to be delayed until January. Harry was depressed because he thought he would have a kidney transplant before Christmas.

The same week his infection was discovered, Les cut off the tip of his middle finger in a sawmill accident. So they both had to heal before the transplant surgery could be done. Christmas came and Harry was happy to be home with his family. In early January, he and Les were both healed, and the date of the transplant was set for January 26, 1972. It was his sister Chris' first birthday.

At this point, Harry was thinking more about his new life to come, and less about what had happened to him. To this day everything that happened to him is a painful subject, and he doesn't like to talk about it. He never realized at the time that he would have to relive the whole thing over again thirty-four years later with his own son.

On January 25, Les and Harry went into the hospital to prepare for the transplant the next day. Harry went on dialysis for what he hoped would be the last time. This operation was life or death to him, because he knew he couldn't live on a dialysis machine for years to come. He sat in his room and listened to the helicopters on the roof possibly bringing in kidneys to other people. He prayed for those people who would also be having a transplant. Harry was a good person and remains so to this day.

The day of the surgery Harry was given very large doses of prednisone. This drug is an immunosuppressive drug given to all transplant patients so that your body won't reject the kidney. He would be taking this and many other pills for the rest of his life. He was wheeled into surgery and he could see his Uncle Les lying on a table across the room. They waved at each other and that is the last thing he remembers until he woke up.

His Mom and John were waiting outside for the operation to be over; it took four hours and was a complete success. They had two patients to take care of. Harry was in ICU for a month. Les was in the hospital a couple of weeks, and then went to stay with Harry's family until he was well enough to go home.

There were some complications at first. Harry and the other patient down the hall who had just had her transplant had a fever and a rejection episode at the same time. They kept them from visiting each other because they wondered if it was related somehow. Things settled down and on February 24, 1972, Harry went home a well man.

No more dialysis, plenty of water to drink, and feeling good at last. He had been in and out of the hospital for six months and not feeling well for a year before that. His only diet restrictions were a low fat, low salt diet. It was really food that everyone should eat; and he kept to it religiously. He was on prednisone, imuran, folic acid, and hygroton, which is a water pill, and phosphagel to coat his stomach and add phosphorus to his diet.

He felt happy and blessed to be the first one to survive kidney disease and be alive in his family. He only wished his Dad could have been saved too.

Harry was told he would always have to come to the Cleveland Clinic for his follow up appointments because they were the only ones who could manage his transplant properly. And if he ever needed any other kind of surgeries, they would have to be done there in order to monitor the transplant.

A short time after he was home, he fell down the stairs and scared himself to death, but he was all right. His hair was also falling out from the large doses of prednisone. The amount of pills would be cut down in time and his hair would grow back.

Harry was going for checkups every two weeks. On March 10, 1972, a friend took Hilda and Harry to Cleveland for his doctor's visit. John had a dentist appointment that morning and then he was going to work. He was so glad to go back after all the time he had missed.

Hilda kept saying that she felt something was wrong. They came home to find John's boss in the living room and everyone crying. Hilda was screaming hysterically by then, running from room to room, calling John's name. He had died of a blood clot to the heart from his dental work while working on the top of scaffolding in Norwalk. Mike and Carol were told that he could have been saved, but the EMS left him up there too long deciding what to do with him. They never told Hilda this.

I don't think Hilda ever

really understood the real reason John died. I think she blamed it on kidney disease, and the stress he had been under driving Harry back and forth to Cleveland and having five more children at home to take care of.

Hilda was alone again to raise three small children by herself. She had never been back to Germany, had never seen her parents again, and now they were gone. There was no one at all to help her. And this is where I came into their lives.

Harry asked me to marry him in the fall of 1973, and I said I needed more time to think about it. I have always regretted that, but I was young and I was scared. Even back then, Harry could only see that he was well and would always be that way. I wasn't so sure. He asked me again on New Years Eve of the same year and I said yes.

It has always been a joke that we must have been drunk when we got engaged. We spent all of our time together. The months went by and we were planned our wedding. It was going to be on October 26, 1974.

CHAPTER THREE

In June of that year, Harry developed a bladder infection, and in those days kidney patients had to go in the hospital so that they could be watched closely. I missed him and would call him every day. I called Hilda on the phone during this time to give her updates. She didn't seem concerned about it at all. To her, this was nothing compared to what she had endured when Harry had his transplant.

I remember vividly sitting in a chair in the living room at my parent's house and the wind was blowing through the windows. I sat there and rocked and thought of the future. Was this what my life was going to be like? Hospitals and sickness? Little did I know that one day this would be true. I was so insecure about all this. I thought myself a coward at the time. Harry was in the hospital a week and then came home.

Sometime before we were married, I went with Harry to one of his appointments at the Cleveland Clinic. I have to say I hated that place from the first moment I saw it. It scared me, but of course, everything did at the time. We went and talked to Harry's nephrologist, who was a kidney doctor and asked him if he thought that this disease might be hereditary. He said there were a lot of people who had this disease and there was no one else in their family who had it. He said that it probably wasn't. I really didn't believe him.

At work, they didn't approve of us both working there. They were starting to make it tough on Harry, and things started to turn ugly there. He had to work a lot of nights until after midnight. He made box designs for the salesmen to take to the clients. They had to be redone over and over to make the customers happy. He never was paid any overtime for all the extra hours he put in. So, a month before we got married, he found another job in a dental lab with some guys I had gone to school with.

My Mom and Dad, Curly Koelsch were planning our wedding. My Dad's real name was Norman, but everyone called him Curly because of his hair. My sister Amy was going to be my maid of honor.

I discussed the fact that Harry had kidney disease in his family with my parents and friends. My mother thought that the disease seemed to run in the men in the family, so she hoped we would have girls. My Dad said Harry and I were just alike and we would be happy together.

In the fall of that year my great grandmother, Anna Walborn had to go into a nursing home. She was 93, and had lived with her daughter, my grandmother Ethel Uhl, for fifty years and she was getting too much to handle. She was such a sweet woman and I loved her dearly. She was heartbroken that she had to go, but she kept falling down.

Harry and I went to see her the day before they took her to the nursing home, and she grabbed our hands and told us we were going to have a long and happy life together. I don't know if she said that because she knew I was scared, or if she simply meant it as a good wish. Years later, I would desperately hang onto what she told us that day.

We had rented an upstairs apartment and started moving our furniture in. My uncles and my Dad moved my stuff. Our couch wouldn't fit through the doorway and had to be pulled upstairs over the front porch with pulleys. Everyone was grumbling; my Mother thought we should take it back for a smaller one. It was then I decided that I would not ask anyone to do anything for us again.

Hilda seemed upset when Harry was moving his things out of her house. I thought at the time that she didn't want him to marry me and leave. Now I realize that she had almost lost him, and it was hard to let him go off with someone and hope that they would take good care of him and make him happy.

A week before our wedding, Harry was in a car accident on the way to my house from work; he was daydreaming and ran a stop sign, and hit a van, which propelled him into someone's driveway. He then hit a sports car and ran into the side of a brick house. He strained his back a little and swallowed some glass from his shattered windshield. He said he was totally shocked; one minute he was at the intersection and the next thing he knew he had a mouthful of glass.

When the police came, they told Harry to lie down in the

grass and rest. Harry told him that his future mother in law had a police radio and his fiancée would probably be there soon, so no way was he lying down and scaring us to death. And sure enough, my mother had on her police radio on and was sure it was Harry in the accident and we ran the three blocks to the site of the accident and took Harry to the emergency room. I was so afraid when I saw that wrecked car; I thought he was dead before we ever got the chance to have a life. But Harry was alright, God only knows how.

We had our rehearsal dinner the night before the wedding. We all went to Harry's house to eat after-wards. Hilda made a nice roast beef meal for everyone in the wedding party. Tomorrow was the big day.

Harry and I were married on October 26, 1974. We had a large wedding and were married in the Catholic Church in Sandusky, Ohio.

It was a beautiful fall day, with the sun shining on the colored fall leaves outside. I stood at the altar holding Harry's hand and prayed that our children would not have kidney disease. Hilda was crying her eyes out; I'm sure she thought she would never see the day that Harry was married and well enough to have his own life. My sister Amy was my maid of honor; a friend of Harry's was the best man. My Dad gave me away. He always said Harry and I were a lot alike and he was happy for me.

We went to southern Ohio for our honeymoon, and went through Ripley. Hilda thought this was a terrible place for a honeymoon. It was a mistake to go there since everyone there knew Harry, and the story about his family and kidney disease. They all saw Harry and were thrilled that he was alive and so healthy. I saw what happened to him as something to be afraid of. I always felt people were looking at Harry like he was a lab experiment because kidney transplants were not common at the time. I just did not understand then how miraculous it really was.

We visited some old neighbors of Harry's that had lived across the street. Their mother, Phyllis Myers was a friend of Hilda's, and Harry had played with her kids when he lived in Ripley. We went to the cemetery to see his Dad's grave; and all I could think was that the Greiner's were lying there so peacefully in death, struck down even before the prime of their lives. It was a very sad place.

When we came back from our honeymoon, I found out that a newspaper reporter had taken our picture at the church and had printed it in the newspaper. Under the picture, the caption read, "Harry Greiner, who had a kidney transplant, has gotten married today to the former Cindy Koelsch and is starting a new life." I was mad; I didn't want our wedding to be about a kidney transplant. I have never been the kind of person who liked attention brought to myself anyway. I like to keep in the background.

We started our life together in our upstairs apartment in Sandusky, Ohio. We were very happy together. We were very young and naïve at the time and believed our faith could change the world. We thought that since Harry already had his transplant, he could not pass this disease on. There wasn't any information on this at the time that we could read about, so we believed what we wanted. And so we buried our doubts, and started our life together.

In the early years of our marriage, we would go and see Hilda and the kids. I loved to hear stories about her life in Germany. I was into genealogy long before it became popular. I would listen to the stories my Great Grandmother told of her childhood when I was only eleven years old.

Harry, Hilda, Nancy and Norma

would all talk about their early years in Ripley. And one strange thing came out of these conversations that none of them had ever told each other before. Nancy, Norma and Harry slept upstairs in the same room together when they were small. This was the same room that their Grandpa had slept in when he had lived with them.

This scary thing happened only at night. Harry said he would lie in bed thinking about what he would do the next day. It was so hot at night in the years before air conditioning that it was hard to go to sleep right away anyhow. Especially in Ripley, as the town was surrounded by hills everywhere and there was never a breeze, just a hot stillness.

Anyway, there were little clusters of grapes all over the wallpaper in the hallway coming up the stairs. As he looked at the grapes, they would seem to move just a little closer. He would turn his head away, and then look back and they kept creeping closer and closer. The last time he looked, they came right up to his face and then flew back to the wall.

Harry was so scared he would hide his face behind his hands and peek through his fingers. They would bounce back and forth from his face to the wall making a swishing noise. Then the grapes would hover in front of his face until he fell asleep. This went on for years, and then it stopped. That and the nightmares of something pressing his body down and clawing his back when he was sleeping at night. After they moved out of there, he just thought it was childhood imagination.

Nancy and Norma both said at once that it had happened to them too. They had never even told each other. They said the flower would make swooshing sounds as it drew back and forth. They would close their eyes and when they opened them, it would still be there in front of their faces. They could not believe that they had all seen the same thing and had not told each other, especially when they were all so scared. They said it just became commonplace after awhile and they would just fall asleep.

Harry, however, added to the story by saying that once when he saw the grape cluster in front of his face, there was a rip in the wallpaper. When he got up in the morning, he found the same spot on the wall and it had the same rip in it. Hilda did not put much stock in the story, but I thought she looked nervous. It probably brought to mind the night that Harry's Dad died and the lights went off and on for her and Les.

It was during this time that we decided to write a book. There were not many transplants at the time and we thought it would make an interesting story. The publishers wanted it to be more of a medical story, and we didn't want it to be written that way, so we put it away for a while. The years went by and now I am glad we never published it since we have a lot more to add after thirty-nine years.

After about a year, we got tired of living in the apartment. It was noisy and the girl downstairs would bring all the men she worked with home with her and party all night. Then we started getting cockroaches. The landlord found fifty bags of garbage in the basement that the party girl was storing there. She was evicted and they were going to fumigate the entire house. We didn't want our clothes and furniture smelling like that, so we had to find another place to move into.

Everyone told us we would not find another place that quickly, but we did. We moved to a rented house on a small side street in Sandusky. We had a backyard and were allowed to have a dog, so we bought a German shepherd. It was ok there, but we wanted our own house someday. I was laid off from work shortly after that and went to work for the county Treasurer doing tax forms. The treasurer actually came and interviewed me at my house to see where I lived, to make sure I was acceptable.

The life of a transplant recipient back then was not easy. The insurance companies considered you a risk. Harry had two small life insurance policies and he tried get a larger one. They denied him coverage. He figured by the time they would give him one, they would say he was too old.

The dental lab was having a hard time getting health insurance for him also. There were only ten people working there, so the business wasn't large enough to have a group policy. They finally found a company to insure him, but we had to pay the higher premium since it was technically our fault it was so high.

He was lucky to have this job because employers at the time were wary of hiring him, they didn't understand what a transplant was and if it had any limitations. I guess they thought he might not be reliable and would be off sick all the time.

Harry always took really good care of himself after his transplant. He was careful about everything he did. It was like living with a science experiment that might go bad. His transplant always seemed like a band-aid, something that might come off at any minute, and was not reliable or safe.

But the truth was, he had been through so much and was just so happy with his transplant that he took good care of it, and believed he would never lose it because it was a gift from his uncle and God.

I never understood anything about transplants back then, and truthfully, I didn't really want to know. I never asked him why he acted the way he did, so I made a lot of my own misery. Later in life, I would learn that he was just always meticulous about everything; it was just part of his personality.

We had gotten married only two years after his kidney transplant. He had to take his blood pressure in the morning and at night and write the results on a sheet of paper in a binder the hospital had made up. He also wrote down how he felt that day, any aches and pains and his urine intake and output. His pills were adjusted a lot and then there were the blood test errors.

Twice the Cleveland Clinic told him he had hepatitis, because someone in the blood lab had mixed his blood tests up with another person. Consequently, Harry always had to consult with other doctors in other departments because of their mistakes. It was scary and frustrating. It didn't seem like a normal life, but it shouldn't have been that way. Instead of repeating the blood test to be sure, the clinic tried to scare you on purpose so you would agree to see more doctors; ergo more money for them. We didn't realize any of this at the time.

Our life started to settle into a normal pattern. Harry changed jobs again. He went to work as a maintenance man for the Catholic Church in our town. We had group insurance for the first time, but what went on there was disgusting. Priests running naked in the parking lot, and one of them was taking high school boys to his cabin in the woods and molesting them.

The priests had pictures of naked women all over their walls, and complained when they had to spend their day off giving someone the last rights. Their basement in the priest house was full of liquor. That was pretty much the end of our belief in the

Catholics.

I was still working for the county treasurer. I hated that job, it was like being with the nuns in the Catholic school, no one was allowed to talk or they got a dirty look. I became so nervous there that I ended up in the hospital. After that, I quit and went to work for a blacktop company in Sandusky typing invoices in their office.

We then decided that we would go to Ripley and visit. I wasn't afraid to go there anymore. I became very interested in the Greiner's and their ancestors. Who they were and what their lives were like. We visited a lot of Harry's old friends. There were people who had known his grandparents, and said his Grandpa had been called Doc Greiner though we never did figure out why. I always wanted Harry to find his Aunt Nancy who had been married to his Uncle Herman. Nobody we asked ever seemed to know where she was.

We saw David Gast, his old childhood friend, and then went on to Seaman, Ohio to visit his Uncle Les. He and his wife Jewell were really happy to see us. I think it did Les' heart good to see Harry so healthy. Les had three kids of his own by then. Les told us stories about his brothers and I wish now I had listened better.

Hilda never wanted to talk about them at all. She always made them sound like drunks that spent all their time in bars. Years later, we would learn that she was there with them. There was not much else to do in a small farm town. She always wanted to make them sound bad, I guess because she was mad that they had all died. This way she could pretend that she didn't care.

When we came back, we found out that Harry's sister Carol was pregnant. She and her husband Mike had a baby boy in 1978 and they named him Jonathan. Chris and Kelley who were Harry's youngest sisters, used to come and stay with us. It seemed odd that they were only seven and eight years old, and they were aunts. They were more like Jon's friends.

In 1979, I was pregnant with our first child. We were thrilled to death. Carol was also pregnant again. One day we got a call that Carol had lost the baby because her blood pressure was too high. She found out she had kidney disease. A horrible feeling of dread came over me. I could feel the baby moving inside me and it was supposed to be a happy time, but it was again clouded over with kidney disease.

I am sure Carol felt the same way about her baby. It was a little boy. Again, we talked ourselves into believing that a transplant would cure the spread of the disease. It was the only way I could calm myself down. Our son Mike was born on April 4, 1980.

We lived in the house for

another year. The country was soon in a recession and there weren't many good paying jobs. We were tired of Ohio and everything in it. We then decided to move to Denver, Colorado. A friend of Harry's from Ripley lived out there and found us a house to rent.

We had a big sale and sold all our furniture. I really hated doing that because everything was new. Little did I know that it would be more than ten years before I ever owned anything new again. My aunt and uncle took us home to eat the night we left. My parents were too busy. My best friend Dee Dee Wensink came to say goodbye. She was pregnant with her first baby and I hated leaving her. We had been the best of friends since we were six years old.

So in the summer of 1981, we headed west with a one year old baby and a German Shepherd dog in the car with us. We had an old

Ford LTD and towed a trailer behind us. We drove straight through and slept in the car.

A strange thing happened on the way there. We turned off one of the turnpike exits in Kansas and were going to pull over to sleep awhile. The exit ended on a country road with a cornfield. A man in a police uniform with a flashlight was standing on the edge of the field. He stopped us and asked where we were going. We didn't see his police car anywhere. He told us we could pull down the road and sleep for a while. It was so eerie that we didn't trust him and got right back on the road. I don't think he was a cop; he probably would have robbed us and maybe even killed us. It was like something out of a horror movie. It gives me goose bumps to this day when I think about it.

We arrived at the house with the brakes gone on the car. Right away we had expenses. We left with dreams in our head. But the reality was that we had to find a job, a bank, a doctor, and a mechanic. We had a year old baby and no insurance. We either had guts or were plain stupid.

We spent the first night there sleeping on newspapers on a dirty living room floor. I just cried, and was so sorry we had come there.

Life was tough out there. The house was old and ugly and very depressing, but in a good neighborhood. The only furniture we had brought with us was our beds. There were jobs, but they all paid minimum wage unless you happened to be in the oil business. I was very homesick for something familiar. We were running out of food and money while Harry looked for a job. We ended up on food stamps and welfare. I had never been so poor in my entire life. We didn't come there very prepared.

Harry worked for a tool

company and several other places. The people were different there than they were in Ohio. They were from a lot of different places and cultures.

Harry finally got a job with a nondenominational church as a groundskeeper. There were really nice people there. We finally made some friends. One of the women we met there brought us bags of groceries one day because we didn't have anything to eat. It was the nicest thing anyone has ever done for us. I didn't feel like I could ask anyone back home for help.

Other people gave us things like a couch and a chair. We ate on a card table. I sure missed my new washer and dryer, especially with having a one-year-old child. We never had any dressers; we kept our clothes in boxes. I just felt so out of place there. We had no money to do what other people did. We couldn't go out to eat. We bought clothes at the thrift store. The old Ford Ltd finally gave out and we didn't have a car. Harry would ride a bike or take the bus to work. I couldn't go anywhere. We used the church truck to get groceries.

We met up with a guy from the box company in Sandusky Harry designed some boxes on the side for him. I worked all kinds of part time jobs, but we never had any money. I had to work at "Burger King" at night, and I had to walk to work because the car didn't run anymore. I would walk the six blocks there and I carried a can of mace with me so when I walked home in the dark I would feel safe. Once while I was working there some guy came in and robbed the place. I had to give him all the money from the cash registers. It was a scary place out there.

Someone heard that we didn't have a car and said he had a Chevy nova, but it was in Kentucky. We could have it if we went there and got it. They gave Harry the money to fly out there and a credit card in case the car needed repairs. The brakes were bad on the car and Harry didn't feel right using that man's credit card, so he drove it back that way. That was a mistake to risk your life that way. All he had to eat was some snacks in the car on the way back. I was so worried about him. Finally after a week, he came back home. I was so glad to see him; I flew out the door and down to the curb and threw my arms around him.

The first time Mike was sick, the doctor wouldn't see him because we had no insurance. Finally, he agreed, and we paid him five dollars a week on the bill. We could hardly afford that. It was pathetic. Thank God, we never got sick.

In 1983 I was pregnant with our second child. We couldn't really afford to have another baby, but we didn't want to wait forever either. We wanted our kids to be close in age so that they could play with each other. If it was a boy, we were going to name him Bob after Harry's Dad. I continued to work at night at "Burger King" until I couldn't fit into my uniform anymore.

Our baby was going to be delivered by midwives, a new program at the hospital. Our friends wanted me to have the baby at home, but I wanted to go to the hospital. Thank God I did. The baby was born three weeks early. When I went into labor, and was examined, I had a tear in my placenta. The baby was surrounded in blood.

Joe was born on September 30, 1983. As soon as he was born, the midwife grabbed a tube and sucked the blood out of his nose with her own mouth so that he could breathe. They took me to a room, and Harry followed them with Joe to an intensive care room. In writing this story, Harry told me that Joe turned a dark purple and almost died. I never knew that at the time, but it still made me cry.

As the midwife was sucking on a tube with her mouth to clear the blood out of Joe's lungs, Harry was begging God to let Joe live. That woman saved our baby's life that night and we are forever grateful.

They put Joe in an oxygen tent that looked like a cake plate cover. They wheeled me down to see him, but I was so weak, I could only sit there a minute. I lay in my room and prayed he wouldn't die. I was so scared. I never even got to hold him. Nine hours later, I knew he would be all right. Harry said that because of what almost happened, he could not name our baby Bob; it just reminded him of a name on a tombstone. We decided to name him Joe after my paternal grandfather.

So now we had two sons. I told Mike he had a new baby brother to play with. I laughed when he said Joe didn't look like he could play with him, all he did was lay around all day. After Joe was born, we wanted to leave Denver and go back to Ohio. Nothing good had ever happened there.

What we failed to see when we moved there was that even though we were miles away from everyone we knew, you cannot run away from yourself. We had been there three years. Harry's mother said she wouldn't help us, she said she didn't tell us to go there in the first place. My Dad wanted us to come back, so we went back home to live with my parents in Sandusky. My sister Amy and her husband had moved to Florida a couple of years before.

We started back east in March of 1984, with a giant snowstorm chasing us across the country and we got home the day before it hit. Everything seemed so small and strange at home. Even our parents looked a lot older. The next day some of my cousins came to see us. It was good to be back. It was not easy for anyone with the four of us moving in after I had been away from home for ten years. And also with the kids being so young; Joe was four months old, and Mike was three.

CHAPTER FOUR

After we had been there eight months, we moved to Milan, Ohio because they had good schools there. We rented this rickety old farmhouse, because it was all we could find in the school district at the time.

The fuel oil furnace and electric water heater were in the basement. There were huge holes in the foundation down there, all the heat escaped out, and the field rats came in. There was no heat in the upstairs at all. We used kerosene and electric heaters to keep warm. If it was too cold, we all slept in the living room on the floor.

The person who owned our

house sold motorcycles and satellite dishes, and Harry got a job working there. One day in 1985, while Harry was unloading a motorcycle, the other guy let it fall and Harry broke the bicep tendon in his arm. The doctor told him that it was better left as it was, because surgery would pull the muscle too tight, and he wouldn't be able to use his arm. He couldn't work for a few months and had to go on worker's compensation. The landlord never lifted a finger to help us; he would not even plow the snow out of our driveway. He was obviously mad that Harry had claimed workmen's compensation.

After that, Harry wouldn't work for him anymore and got a different job. He had several small jobs and finally got a state job working in the maintenance grounds department. I had several part time jobs, and finally decided that I would clean offices at night so I could stay home with the kids during the day.

One of the jobs I had was selling shoes in a department store. Harry's sister Norma worked there too. She came to work one day and told me she had just found out she had kidney disease. I was really upset, as if somebody had kicked me in the heart. Of course, Nancy's kidneys failed soon after that since they were twins. Hilda was indifferent to the whole thing, but I knew she was upset. She just looked like she expected it to happen.

Norma was married by then, and went on home peritoneal dialysis. You hooked up to a machine at night through a tube in your stomach. The dialysis machine went through all the cleaning cycles while you slept and was done in the morning. That way you could still work. Nancy was also on this type of dialysis.

Norma developed peritonitis one time while she was on dialysis. You have to be very sterile with the tube in your stomach or you can possibly get an infection in your peritoneal cavity. Both Nancy and Norma were on the waiting list for a kidney. A couple of years later, Norma got a call for a kidney. She went to the Cleveland Clinic. She had the kidney transplant and everything seemed fine at first.

Hilda didn't want to go to the hospital anymore for the transplant surgeries. I couldn't understand at the time how you would not go to the hospital when your own child was having such serious surgery. I don't think she could stand it. Myself, I didn't want to hear anything about it. I was too scared and tried to hide from it. I'm sure they probably thought I seemed somewhat heartless.

After a couple of weeks, Norma started feeling sick. She was admitted to the hospital. The Cleveland Clinic had given her a kidney with a blood clot in it and the kidney was failing. After several weeks of worthless testing the kidney was taken out. Of course, the clinic called it a rejection. We have found from talking to other people that they generally call it that when anything goes wrong with a transplant. You never get the real reason, especially when it is their fault.

At the same time Norma lost her kidney, her husband left her. It was very cruel to decide to leave her when she was so sick and in the hospital. Naturally, she was very depressed. Do you think the Cleveland Clinic understood this? They never even bothered to try.

Then they gave her some kind of medicine that was making her talk incoherently. Instead of finding out what was wrong, they decide they are going to transfer her to the mental ward. Another department and more money. If they put you in there, you have a very hard time getting back out. Carol and Nancy went up there and saved her from that fate.

You cannot be left alone at that place; you never know what will happen to you. If the nurses and doctors on the hospital floor that you are on would take responsibility to solve what is wrong with you there, these things wouldn't happen.

Instead, they just move their patients around like cattle and let somebody else worry about it. The patient's real problem gets lost in the shuffle, many times resulting in death.

When Norma came home from the hospital, I was shocked at her appearance. She looked just like someone who had been in a concentration camp. She was pale, thin and extremely weak. God only knows what they did to her in there in those couple of weeks. So she was back on dialysis and the transplant list. Within the next year, Nancy had her transplant and Norma had hers shortly afterward.

By then I just got used to everyone in this generation having kidney disease. I still thought that maybe it would not affect our kids. Harry's Dad had the disease when his kids were born, so we thought that maybe that is why they all had it. It was just a form of denial.

Harry would get upset with me every time another family member got the disease. I would get all riled up again. He still did not believe it would happen to our kids. I wanted the kids to have blood tests done to have peace of mind. Harry said it was like playing the lottery and knowing you are never going to win. I realized it would just scare the kids anyway, and I did not want that just to make me feel better. And, what would we do anyway if we knew? It would just prey on our mind until the time came, which in this family is in your twenties. I didn't want to relive Hilda's life.

Every holiday there was always a story about kidney transplants. Could there be another subject? I just wished we could talk about something else. I was always trying to find a reason for everybody having kidney disease, and they just accepted it as something natural. They didn't care why. But I had two kids to worry about and they didn't.

It was time for Mike to start kindergarten. He told me the first day, "I am not going to like it here, but I guess I am going to have to go." He was such a logical little boy, and true to his word, he hated the whole twelve years of school.

When Mike was in the second grade, the kids came down with the chicken pox. Harry's doctor at the Cleveland Clinic told Harry he thought he should stay away from the kids until they were well. He told Harry he thought he could possibly get shingles from the chicken pox virus because of the immunosuppressive pills he took, and he would have a hard time getting rid of them. Harry could not even change the kid's diapers after they had their baby shots either because of the chance of picking up the virus they were inoculated against.

His doctor told us to call the infectious disease department at the clinic. In our opinion, he should have talked to them himself and advised Harry what to do. But Harry was left trying to explain his concerns to someone at a desk in a department who obviously knew absolutely nothing about kidney transplants, and he wasn't even their patient. Their motto was, let someone else worry about it. We might as well have asked someone down the street for all the help he got.

He didn't want to take any chances, so Harry moved in with his mother and sisters in Norwalk. My mother did not want him staying at their house, which would have been more convenient since he worked in Sandusky. Harry bought cans of food and vegetables and ate them for supper; no one offered to cook him anything and he didn't want to bother anyone.

He had to work his job all day, and clean offices for me at night, so I could stay with the kids. Harry's sisters could not help me either since they also had kidney transplants. There was no one to help us out.

Joe was really sick and feverish with the chicken pox, and cried continually. He had spots over every inch of his body and was so miserable. It was time for Halloween and I asked my Mom to take Mike trick or treating. They didn't stay out very long because it was suppertime and Mom wanted to get home. Mike was disappointed he didn't get to go to more houses.

On Thanksgiving Day, I sat down and cried because I was all alone. Hilda told me she would have another turkey dinner when we could all be together. She knew how depressed I was and told me "this too shall pass." Harry would come over and talk to me through the screen door. We sure did miss each other.

He had to wait until all the scabs came off the kids before he could come home. I scrubbed down the entire house after the kids were well. It was two months before Harry was able to come home.

We lived in that house for a couple of years until the landlord said he wanted to sell it, so we started looking for something else. We found another house in Milan that was smaller, but we could be warm and it had central air conditioning. This was the best house we had lived in. The kids had friends and could go down the street and play.

It was time for Joe to start school, and how he hated it. He was so close to me and cried everyday he had to go. I would go by the school and watch him on the playground at recess. He would be sitting on the bench by himself. It broke my heart to see him there. He was like that for two years before he got used to it. I was the same way when I went to school. Oddly enough, he would be the one who had all the friends later on and loved school.

In the spring of 1989, I got a call to come to the hospital; Harry had been taken there by ambulance from work. They told me they thought he had hurt his back. I sat in the emergency room with his clothes in a bag waiting for some news. It wasn't his back, his quadriceps tendon had ripped off his kneecap, it was rolled up in the top of his leg, and he couldn't walk. They said he would have to have surgery to repair the tendon.

Believe it or not, we still believed the crap that the Cleveland dished out that you had to have surgery there to have your transplant monitored. The clinic always said that small towns had hillbilly hospitals and were not equipped to take care of kidney patients. We even had to go all the way to Cleveland for blood work. Really, they just wanted all the money for themselves.

I couldn't go; the kids were little and there was no one to leave them with. My parents were in Florida at my sister's house. So, Nancy and Norma came and took Harry to Cleveland. The first mistake the hospital made was putting Harry on the kidney floor instead of the orthopedic one.

I went there the day of the surgery with Norma. We sat in this huge waiting room with what seemed like hundreds of people. They would call out your name when the surgery was over. It was like a cattle call and it seemed to go on forever. When Harry got back to his room, he was in terrible pain. He just kept hitting that morphine button. Norma and I had to go home and go to work. I really hated leaving him there. At that time, I still believed he would be okay there by himself.

In the morning I called and he was no better. The so called doctors on call at night, who are in reality the students, had come in and said there was nothing they could do until morning when the orthopedic doctors came on call.

They are so worthless there at night. Half of them do not speak English and the other half knows nothing. They might as well close down the hospital at night. The doctors there are supposedly specialists. However, they know nothing about other parts of the body except their own specialty, if you are lucky enough for them to know that much.

That is only one of their huge problems. Most people that are in a hospital have a variety of medical problems and since the doctors from different departments refuse to work with each other because they are too arrogant, the patient ends up suffering the consequences. Your other medical problems are overlooked and you sometimes pay with your life. So much for their "teamwork" that that they so heavily advertise.

I felt so helpless. Harry had been in pain all night. I called the ombudsman office; a place in the hospital that you can take your complaints to. I didn't know at the time what a joke that place was. They are not there to help you; they are only a buffer for the doctors and the hospital.

Later that morning they finally figured out that the bandage on his leg was wound too tight, and because of that, it was pulling the incision apart. That's what you get when interns are allowed to "learn" in the operating room. Twenty-four hours of constant pain just because of that. What morons and total incompetence! After a couple of days, he came home.

Well, it was a rough time. Harry had to be helped to do everything. Going to the bathroom, getting dressed; the whole nine yards. That of course goes along with this kind of surgery. I had to get someone to drive us to Harry's doctor's appointments in Cleveland; I wasn't used to driving in big cities.

Harry had been walking down a ramp at work when he broke his tendon, so he was eligible for worker's comp. The place he worked at was fighting that even though it had happened there. We had to get a workman's comp lawyer to fight the case.

Then of course, the Cleveland Clinic took months to fill out the paperwork he needed. They don't care if you don't have any money to live on. You have to badger them to get anything done. Everybody seemed to be holding us back from getting our benefits. It is bad enough to be off work and need surgery without all this other crap going on.

The night before Easter Sunday, something happened to Harry's cast. It somehow turned around on his leg and was pushing his knee in and causing pain. We called the clinic and no one could help him until Monday morning. No one in town would help you either if you were a patient at the Cleveland Clinic; the feeling being that since they did the surgery they should take care of it. They pretty much know around here how much the clinic screws up and they don't want to be responsible for it.

Well, we were on our own as usual and what do you do if you are in excruciating pain and no one will help you? He cut the cast off himself, and bound his leg with metal supports until the next morning.

When we got to Cleveland, we waited three hours in the waiting room for the doctor. We were told that one of the players from the Cleveland Browns was in the office and they were the doctor's first priority. He was the orthopedic doctor for the Cleveland sports teams and he thought that made him important.

When we finally got in there, the doctor took one look at Harry's homemade cast and said insultingly, "I could fire you as a patient for cutting off that cast." Harry told him "I could fire you as a doctor since the clinic refused to help me over the weekend." The doctor was an arrogant son of a bitch anyway. Harry was sent to have his leg recast and we went back home.

Joe was in the second grade and it was time for him to make his first communion. We were still trying to do the right thing for our kids at the time even though we didn't believe in the Catholic Church anymore. We were still somewhat undecided at that time about what to do about the kids as far as their religious training. Harry always claimed that Mike only wanted to go to CCD because they gave out candy bars.

Harry couldn't go to church for Joe's first communion because he couldn't get around well enough. I was really disappointed. My Mom and Dad came and went with the kids and I, and we had a small party afterwards.

The day finally came when Harry could get his cast taken off, and his leg was frozen stiff. It didn't seem like it would ever bend again. The clinic made him come there for physical therapy, which really was ridiculous. Consequently, he did not get the care he should have had because the clinic was so far away from where we lived. They let him do some of the exercises at home.

Harry has always been self sufficient when it comes to taking care of himself, but it sure made it harder on him. He had to decide how far he could push that leg without hurting it, and he did a good job. So, day by day he had to exercise his leg to get it to move. The clinic never wants to let go of any money, so they won't let you do anything in your own town.

After six months, the clinic decides he can go back to work. His leg was still very weak and he was a groundskeeper. The clinic refused to sign any papers for him to be off any longer. So he went back to work limping. It was rough for Harry trying to do his job. The doctors have no idea what a normal person does for a living, and they never listen or consider the patient or what is best for them.

After a while, Harry's leg strengthened back up and things finally got back to normal. Harry did everything for the kids. He never ever got over losing his Dad at such a young age. He told me stories of the other kids having their Dad's and he never had one.

Hilda would never talk about him at all. I guess it was just too painful. Harry is upset about it to this day.

We made sure the kids led normal lives. We camped out with them, had birthday parties; all the things kids do. Mike looked like me and Joe was the splitting image of his Dad, which made me worry that he would be the one who would have kidney disease.

This is very sad since you should be proud when your children look like you. I was just always obsessed with the fear of it. You should not be able to predict your child's future. You should be thinking about what they will be when they grow up, not what disease they will have.

In 1992, three years after he broke his quad tendon, Harry was carrying a desk at work and the other person dropped their end. He broke the bicep tendon in his opposite arm near his elbow. I thought, here we go again. We had to wait a month for an appointment at the Cleveland Clinic, so he had to be off work with his arm in a sling waiting. If he had another type of job, he could have worked while he was waiting to see the doctor.

When we finally went to have Harry's arm looked at, he was told he needed to have surgery again to repair the tendon. It was scheduled for three weeks later. This one would be outpatient surgery.

The day of the surgery, my parents went with us. Harry was sitting in the pre-surgery room waiting. Someone came up to check his wristband to take him to surgery. My mother overheard them saying something about prostate surgery. If she had not said something, God only knows what would have happened. They had him mixed up with an eighty-year-old man who was going to have prostate surgery. The other man was already in the operating room, so they had to take him out and sanitize the room again to make it sterile and switch the two patients. They are so utterly incompetent it is unbelievable.

Harry was going to stay awake for the surgery, which was an option they gave him. The surgeon's assistant, which was of course a student, could not get the needle in right to numb his arm. The other two students were begging to try, and after three failed attempts, they had to put him under.

Six hours later, we were on our way home. I hate it when they discharge you like that. Harry was on Tylenol III and all incoherent sitting on the couch staring at his arm as if he just could not figure out why there was a cast on it. That was a very long night, needless to say.

The kids were pretty much depressed to see their Dad injured again. It was Mike's twelfth birthday and it wasn't much fun.

Harry was pretty much incapacitated again, but he had physical therapy in our hometown this time. We refused to go back and forth to Cleveland for this. They didn't like that at all. Time went on and Harry went back to work again.

Hilda was diabetic and had several strokes. She was in the hospital and was put on a lot of pain medication. She kept saying that she had to carry the bottles of blood down the hall. I realized she was remembering the time that Bob, Harry's Dad had been on dialysis and they made her carry the bottles of his blood to where they had taken him down the hall. Evidently, this nightmare had stayed with her always. That story always sounded gruesome to me and I felt so bad for her.

Around this same time the kids starting asking questions about kidney disease in the family, and wondered if they would have it too. I would say it wasn't likely;

I didn't want their childhood ruined like Harry's was. And I didn't know for sure anyway.

The company that Harry had life insurance with finally told us they thought they could get him a bigger policy. He only had a twenty five hundred dollar policy from when he was a kid. He had a physical and they gave him a fifty thousand dollar policy, but he had to pay a higher rate because of his age and his transplant. It kind of made us mad that they acted as if they were doing him a really big favor.

During this time, Hilda had someone staying with her that was getting a divorce. His ex wife worked with Harry. When Hilda tried to interfere with Harry's job over this, a big fight started and the family took opposite sides and everyone went their separate ways. It was really a shame. We never talked to any of them for years afterward.

Then the house we were living

in had problems with the leach bed and the septic tank in the backyard. The toilet would back up in the bathtub, so we couldn't use the toilet most of the time. The landlord couldn't afford to fix it right away. We threatened him with the health department, and he finally had it fixed. We didn't want to take the kids out of the school system, and houses in that area were hard to find, so we stuck it out.

We had gotten money for partial disabilities over the years because Harry's leg and arms were never quite the same. We almost had enough money for a down payment on a house. We were getting so sick of living in other people's houses. We wanted to paint the walls the color we wanted and do what we wanted with the yard. The neighbors always looked down on us because we were the renters. Mike was going to start high school and Joe junior high. We wanted to stay in Milan because of the schools, so we started looking for a house.

We had a realtor showing us houses and he was losing his patience with us. We were looking for a house to suit us and hadn't found it yet. He said our kids would be out of school before we found a house to please us.

We found a house we wanted to see on a private drive in Norwalk; it was still in the Milan school district. We called another realtor to show it to us. It was on a private drive with a stone roadway. The house was built in 1966 and had a huge pond in the backyard. We knew this was the one. We finally had our own house; we were so excited!

The woman who had owned the house had already moved out. Her husband had died in the house and she couldn't stand to live there. We had a month before we had to move out of the rented house so we had a lot of time to paint and get things ready to move in. It makes me sick to think how full of hope

we were for this house. We thought
we were leaving all of our bad
memories behind. Little did we
know the worst ones were yet to
come.

CHAPTER FIVE

We moved in January of 1995. The kids could both have their own rooms now. Harry and I started remodeling the house that first winter. We could finally have everything the way we wanted it.

The first summer we lived there, Harry decided he would build a cabin for the kids to camp out in. He had always wanted to do something like this for the kids and was excited that they could build this together.

He started it the first day of their summer vacation. That was his first mistake; they wanted to go with their friends, not spend the summer building a cabin. Mike was the one who ended up staying to help his Dad. When it was done, the kids ended up resenting their Dad for making them work, and Harry ended up with very hurt feelings because they didn't want to do this with him.

He wanted to do something for them that he never could do on rented property and I guess it was just a few years too late. Mike and Joe were not interested in it anymore. They only slept in it a couple of times and now it's a storage shed and a bad memory.

The first few years we were really happy there. Then after awhile you could just feel the tension in the air. Harry spent every living minute working on the house. This was the first and only house we had ever owned. I was in menopause and was not an easy person to live with. And the kids, now that they were teenagers, were also starting to be a handful.

Harry just could not understand why the kids didn't have more respect for us. He had never had a father and thought they should appreciate having one. I told him that this is something that kids should expect to have, and that they have no idea what it would be like for him to be gone and I didn't want them to know. I think after awhile he came to understand that. We had always had a good marriage, but we were starting to have a lot of arguments.

Mike kept telling us stories that he heard someone walking up the stairs at night when we were all asleep. He was always awake late at night. Then he started hearing a man and woman whispering in the hallway. He thought it was Harry and I, but when he opened our door, we were asleep.

Shortly after that, Joe started starting to play his radio all the night long and irritating everyone. He always had to have noise going at night to sleep. Years later, we found out he did it to block out the people talking in the hallway. He would never admit at the time that he heard them too.

I had actually heard the footsteps on the stairs one night and it scared me to death. Sometimes, I would be in the basement washing clothes, and would hear someone walking around upstairs. I thought one of the kids were up since they always slept late, but when I checked they were still asleep.

Harry thought it was a lot of nonsense, which I thought odd, because he had had similar experiences when he was a kid. I think he just thought that since Mike and I watched all those scary movies we were imagining things. After the woman who had lived here died, the voices just stopped. We just all assumed that maybe her husband was looking for her since he died in the house, and now she was with him.

In the spring of 1998, I was at home during the day and I heard the garage door open downstairs and Harry had come home early from work. He was holding his arm and I just stood there and stared at him, and thought "now what?" He said he was afraid to come home and tell me he hurt his arm again. He knew from experience he had broken the bicep tendon in his other arm, because the muscle was just hanging down. I just could not believe it; every three years for the last twelve years he had some orthopedic injury and I was getting paranoid and extremely superstitious.

The prognosis for this arm was the same as the other, no surgery or the muscle in his arm would be too tight to use. The rules at his job had changed, so he was able to go back to work with his arm in a sling and do light duty work until it healed. At least there was to be no surgery and that was a relief. Eventually his arm was healed and life moved on again.

Mike was very good at art, and when he was a sophomore in high school, he won the contest for the best drawing for the Thomas Edison bicentennial in Milan. His drawing was on all the banners they hung in the town square. He was on the evening news and got his picture taken with the Thomas Edison impersonator they hired for the event. It was a special day for all of us.

The years went by and Mike was a senior, he was shy and had one or two good friends, and couldn't wait to get out of school. He graduated in the spring of 1999. Joe was a freshman and had a lot of friends, and was always burning the candle at both ends. He had a lot of flu's, colds and sinus infections, and when he got sick, he was down for the count.

He never seemed to be able to get over any sickness without antibiotics and extra care. Mike was always more healthy. I blamed myself, I thought I hadn't taken very good of care of myself when I was pregnant with Joe. We had lived in Denver at the time, and had very little food to eat.

After Mike graduated, he went to work in a drug store in Huron, Ohio. He was nineteen now, and his cholesterol was slightly high, so he started having blood tests. I asked our family doctor to have kidney function tests done at the same time. Mike was nineteen and getting close to the age that some of our family members had developed kidney disease.

I sweated bullets the couple of days of waiting for the results, but they came back normal. I was encouraged by this because you can detect this type of kidney disease as early as age six, and if there was no sign of it by then we were doing good. He had the same tests for the next six years and they were always normal. Thank God!

I was still worried about Joe getting kidney disease. He looked so much like Harry! I walked into his room one day, and looked over at the wall beside his bed. I swore I could see a dialysis machine sitting there on a small table. I felt like I was in a trance. I shook myself out of it and just stared at the wall. I was scared it was a premonition, and hoped it was just the anxiety I always had about it.

Several years passed and we were still working on the house. Harry, trying to give us everything he never could, spent so much time on the house that he ended up ignoring us. By the time he made time to do something with the kids, they were too old and were off with their friends. We all just drifted farther apart.

In the fall of 2000, Joe came home sick and had an excruciating headache. I took him to the doctor and she thought he might have viral meningitis. We were so upset. We had to go to the hospital so Joe could have a spinal tap, and it came back positive. I was so scared I felt like fainting on the floor until they said it was the non-fatal type.

Joe had to be admitted to the hospital, and he threw up constantly for three days until the headache went away. All the nurses came in with masks on for fear he was contagious, even though the doctor said he wasn't. Joe's school had some concerns about whom he had come in contact with before he got sick.

Of course, Harry had to stay away because he took immuno-suppressant drugs and he couldn't take the chance of getting meningitis. I stayed day and night at the hospital; I didn't want to leave Joe and I didn't know if I was going to get meningitis also, so I stayed away from Harry.

And let me tell you, Joe is not a good patient. He can get

really nasty; he hates hospitals and being sick. Harry and Mike sanitized the house and we brought Joe home after a week. He was out of school about a month; it took him awhile to get his strength back. Harry and I were so thankful to God that Joe came through all right. Joe had always been the one to give us medical scares, but nothing like what was to come.

That winter was uneventful, but in the spring my mother called to tell us she had cancer in her left kidney, and that she would need surgery to remove it. My sister Amy is a nurse and she came home from Florida to stay with Mom. Her surgery reminded me of what it would be like to donate a kidney.

I told my Mom and Dad that I would probably be having a similar surgery someday to donate a kidney to one of my kids. It just brought up all those issues in my mind. The talk was all about living with one kidney. The cancer was encapsulated, so Mom came through all right. Amy stayed another two weeks and went back home.

That spring Harry and I went to see Carol's son Jon. He told us he had gout in his legs and when he went see the doctor about it they told him his kidneys were failing. He was devastated and I knew then that there was no hope that our children would escape this disease.

Harry, forever the optimist, said that Carol had kidney disease when she was pregnant with Jon and maybe that was how it was passed on. Harry was the only one to have kids after having a kidney transplant. Again, we managed to talk ourselves out of believing it could happen to our kids.

Mike I had hope for because his blood tests were always good. Joe was going into his senior year of high school, and I was scared for him. I went into denial again, but deep down I knew better.

In June, Harry and I decided to get our financial affairs in order. We made out a will and were looking into getting more insurance. We filled out an application at our local insurance company, and our agent told up he would need Harry's medical records to file the claim because of his kidney transplant.

Well, after a month and a half of trying, the insurance agent just could not get the Cleveland Clinic to send those records. I tried myself to get them, but it was just like a brick wall of ignorance. It became clear that the clinic was just not going to give them to us. They are so incompetent. Because of them, the life insurance form was never filed, and he didn't get the insurance. But what was to happen next in our life made this insignificant.

Toward the end of July of 2001, Harry started having a pain below his ribs. I was worried and this went on for several weeks. On the evening of August 6, Harry fell asleep on the couch; he had been so tired for several days. It was a strange night; the sky and trees outside had a sick looking greenish yellow tint to them. When I looked out the window, I thought it looked like the end of the world, and it just added to my anxiety. I kept asking Harry if he was alright, and he just brushed it off.

The next night I had to work. Harry and I were talking about how the Cleveland Clinic was not sending his records for the insurance policy. He just said, "It will work out, we have time, after all what could happen?" Famous last words.

I got home from work that night an hour and a half early, and that was unusual. I found Harry lying on the couch upstairs unable to move. Mike and Joe were with their friends. Harry had been lifting weights and pulled a muscle in his chest; he crawled up the stairs and couldn't make it any farther than the couch.

I didn't think it was just a pulled muscle, and I wanted to call the rescue squad. Instead, he tells me to go get his blood pressure cuff. His blood pressure was very low, and I called the rescue squad and they took him to Fisher Titus, the local hospital. I rode in the ambulance with him and I was so scared.

He was taken right in and seen by a nice young doctor there. He was taken for a CAT scan right away, and the vascular surgeon from Sandusky was called. I didn't realize at the time how quickly things were moving along. Later I would see it as a miracle, but not then.

The surgeon came in and told me Harry had an aneurysm in his spleen and he could operate, but people usually never lived through it. I stood there by myself terrified beyond words and stared dumfounded. All I could think was that if there was any chance I had to save that kidney transplant, so I told them to take him to the Cleveland Clinic; my mistake. I should have had him taken to Metro in Cleveland, but I didn't know what I know now.

He had to be life flighted by helicopter and they told me he probably wouldn't make it there because the aneurysm had burst inside him. I looked at Harry and tried to tell him what he meant to me because I thought I was saying goodbye to him. But the words all seemed hollow, what could you possibly say in five minutes that hadn't been said in all our years together? We had been married twenty-seven years at the time.

I called Nancy and Norma, we had been talking to each other again by that time, and Norma came to get me. The life flight came and Norma and I watched it take off with tears in our eyes. By now it was 11:30 at night and we knew we had to get to Cleveland. I didn't even know if Harry would be alive when we got there.

She left me at home to get some things together and get the kids. She went to get Nancy. I ran in the house and Joe was there but I couldn't find Mike anywhere and thought we would have to go without him. He finally came home and we all took off.

The ride there seemed endless, and I was afraid what I would find when I got there. Would he even be alive? It was a horrible nightmare and my stomach was in knots. It was the longest ride I had ever taken and one I will never forget.

When we got there, Harry was alive and was able to talk to us. The nurses at the clinic said the aneurysm hadn't burst, but I found out later they were wrong. It seemed to be taking forever to get the surgery started and Harry was in critical condition. They were waiting for blood in case he needed to have transfusions.

It was 6:00 the next morning before they took him into surgery. Halfway through it, Mike and I were standing in the hallway and the anesthesiologist came out. We asked him what was going on in there and he said it didn't look good; there was blood everywhere and he might not make it.

I will bet any amount of money he was not legally allowed to give us that information. It just terrified us more. I sat that entire time trying to reach out to Harry with my mind, to tell him to hold on. I actually felt like I connected with him at some point. We waited two more hours for the bad news; but he made it through surgery and was in critical condition.

That day was a nightmare of unspeakable emotion that I will never want to relive, but in writing this, I am reliving one of the blackest days of my life. We sat in that ICU waiting room waiting to see Harry. Finally, they let us in to see him for a short time.

There were tubes coming out of him everywhere. His whole body was full of blood, the critical place being in his lungs. He was on a respirator and his skin was deathly white. While we were in there all the receptacles that were connected to the tubes in him were filling rapidly with blood and the nurses shoved us out of the room. His room was right in front of the swinging doors to the ICU, and we could see his cubicle through the glass window in the doors. We saw ten people rush around his bed to start working on him.

I was so tired, petrified, and worn out from worrying that I didn't know which end was up. They said they might have to operate again because they thought blood was leaking somewhere inside him and that he probably wouldn't survive another surgery. Well somehow, that crisis passed, but no one bothered to tell us for another hour.

The kids looked like they couldn't take anymore and they went home with Nancy and Norma. After that, there were a lot more crisis that day as Harry fought for life, and I was there by myself. I just asked myself if this was it, was our life over?

I pretty much thought Harry was going to die that day and where would I tell them to take him. We had never discussed this except that we wanted to be cremated. And for some reason I kept thinking of the nursery window we would never stand at and see our first grandchild; that is if we were blessed with any. I just felt pure terror. I thought of my great grandma and that day long ago when she told us that we would have a long and happy life together. I tried to hold onto that thought.

I had called my Mom and Dad

earlier that day and they were shocked. My Dad offered to come and stay with me, as my Mother was still recovering from her cancer surgery. My cousin brought my Dad later in the day.

The day wore on and on endlessly. At one point, a very dear friend of ours that worked in the clinic came up to ICU to sit with me, and it helped push the terror back for awhile. She told me Harry was good right down to his soul and that he deserved another chance. I will never forget her for coming to offer me comfort on the darkest day of my life.

You were only allowed in ICU certain hours of the day and there was no way I was leaving that hospital. There used to be a big room downstairs with about twenty couches in it where people could sleep. That is gone now and you have to pay to stay somewhere or sleep in a chair.

But that night my Dad and I stayed down there. I was so

exhausted I laid down and my Dad said to me that it was only 9:00 and he never went to sleep until 11:00, as if there was anything remotely normal about where we were. If I wasn't so depressed, I could have laughed at the matter of fact way he said that; but that was my Dad.

I stayed there for a week; my Mom was worried about me staying there alone at night, but I was not leaving. People would come during the day to see Harry and leave at night. All his sisters came; a crisis always brings the family back together. Norma and Joe cried every time they looked at Harry and left the room. I just sat there holding his hand begging him to come back to me.

They had him in a self-induced coma, and he even tried to fight that. I knew how determined he always was to live, and he had always told me he would never leave me, but I thought not even Harry had the will to overcome that set of circumstances.

The main concern was the blood in his lungs. They said Harry might be a on a respirator for a year or more if they could even get his lungs to clear up. He was in critical condition and it was going to take a long time if ever for him to get well again.

The one thing that really scared us is that Harry had blood pouring into his urine bag and we knew this could not be good; but no one would tell us why. The kidney doctors that were on hospital rounds would come and see him and ask me questions about what his creatinine and bun usually ran. These are kidney function tests.

Of course, I knew these answers, but I thought to myself, why are they asking me and don't they have his records up here? They were having a fit over the blood test results, but I myself didn't think his kidney test results were that bad considering

Harry was in critical condition. But why did he have all that blood in his urine?

I asked one of the interns at night if his kidney transplant was doing alright, and all he had to say was, "What good is a kidney transplant without the person? He's in critical condition; we have too many other problems to be concerned about." Well, there's your wonderful bedside manner.

I only knew that he surely wasn't going to make it if he went into kidney failure. And I wondered where Harry's regular doctor was that he had been seeing for twenty years, only to find out that some of the older doctors don't make hospital rounds.

I made a call to his doctor once, be damned the protocol, because they weren't giving Harry all of his kidney medication. The interns in ICU said he didn't need all of them right now, only the prednisone. No way was I going to take their word for it. Finally, someone from his office came to ICU and looked into the matter.

One day Mike and I were sitting in the waiting room and one of the nephrologists walked by, we asked again about the blood in his urine, and he just nonchalantly said it was just the way his body had of getting rid of all the blood that had been spread throughout his body during the surgery. You would think that someone could have told us that when I kept asking about it. It felt like a great weight had been lifted off our shoulders.

Still, I didn't trust the people in there; they would never answer any questions. His heart would race; they put more JP drains in his stomach, and would constantly suck out a substance from his lungs through the respirator. I never knew why they did any of this; it just endlessly worried me. He had three chest ex-rays every day and he never seemed to improve. It was a strain to keep a constant watch on what they were doing when you are not being told everything.

It was nearing the end of August and Joe had to go back to school; it was his senior year. I felt so sorry for him because this should have been a happy time.

Mike took a lot of time off work to go back and forth to Cleveland with me. The stress was making the kids sick, so our doctor had to put them on medicine to relax their stomachs. Mike was only twenty years old with a critically ill father and a mother who was a basket case and it was a lot to handle. I have always protected Joe more, he has always been more fragile and sensitive; but it was not fair to Mike.

One day Hilda called me at the hospital. I had not seen or talked to her in five years, since the day the family had split up over that argument. She really wanted to see Harry, and was half afraid if Harry saw her he would think he was dying. He was in a coma and I doubted that he knew anything. I was not going to be the one to deny her seeing her son since there was a chance he wouldn't live. The last stroke that she had left her in a wheelchair.

Nancy, Norma, Hilda and I went together to Cleveland several days later. Hilda was shocked at his appearance; and she started to cry. I don't know how she could bare to see him that way. Chris, who is Harry's youngest sister, told me that the night Harry was life flighted to Cleveland Hilda just sat at home and kept saying she just couldn't lose her only son.

When we got in the car later, Nancy was saying that it was so hot in there she couldn't breathe. Hilda told her to be quiet and be glad she could breathe at all. Harry was on oxygen and had all that blood in his lungs.

One day when Mike and I got

there, we were told to wait outside, and that made us really nervous because we could see through the door that a group of people were standing around Harry's bed. After an hour, we went in and found out that they had taken out all the wires in his chest and replaced them with new ones. These connected him up to the various machines he was on.

They had let the students do it, and there was blood all over his chest, his hair, his face and on the pillow behind his head. There were curtains between the patients instead of walls, and there was blood all over them too. I wanted them to clean him up, but they were in no hurry.

It was not sterile in there at all. And because of the curtains, you could hear everything being said about the other patients. There was no room to sit down in there either; you had to just stand there for the two hours you were allowed in the cubicle. I had someone tell me later that only the people with money were allowed to sit on chairs in there.

The waiting room for ICU became our home away from home. All the patients' families would wait there between the hours you could go in and visit in the ICU. One man had a laptop and would conduct his business, another woman would knit, and some would be paying bills; whatever you could accomplish while waiting. You soon became friendly with everyone in there.

After awhile, Harry would try to write on a piece of paper to tell us what he wanted to say. The nurses didn't understand why he wasn't in a complete coma with all the medicine they gave him, but he just kept fighting it. And whatever he managed to scribble was complete nonsense, and he seemed upset that we couldn't understand. One coherent thing he managed to write was to leave and let him die. Mike was the only one

148

to see it and kept it from me. The poor kid really carried a load on his shoulders.

By now, I was going home every night because I had to work or I wouldn't get paid. I had a pager and my cell phone and they never left my side, I was so afraid they would call and tell me Harry had died. I would call the ICU at 10:00 every night to make sure he was alright, and then the first thing in the morning before I left for Cleveland.

Home soon became a terrifying place for me, I was afraid Harry would never come back. I hated to even look at the fireplace mantel because I imagined I would see a funeral urn sitting on it one day soon. Mike and Joe had a lot to handle with me being the way I was.

Mike and I would sit by the hours trying to analyze what was said to us in the ICU, what it meant, and then tried to talk ourselves into believing that

Harry would be alright. We just drove ourselves crazy, but it was the only way we could survive. Mike would try to comfort me when I cried and was afraid that Harry would never come home again. It was really too much of a burden for him, but I have always loved and appreciated him for that.

One night after work, I was afraid to go home and face the emptiness, so I went rushing madly into my parent's house. I started crying, saying that Harry would never get well again. My Dad, always the optimist, told me he could see Harry coming back there and sitting in the chair he always sat in. I wanted so badly to believe that. I felt a little better after that.

A few days later, my Mom and Dad took us to Cleveland to see Harry. Mom couldn't stay long because she was still so weak from her own surgery. While we were there, the machines hooked up to Harry's heart monitor started going all crazy, and they said his heart was beating too fast. Everyone was running around beside his bed again, so Mike and I decided to stay until we knew he was alright again. There was always a crisis going on and you never knew what would happen one day to the next. Carol came back that night and took us home.

The next week, Harry was running a fever and they said he had pneumonia. The infectious disease doctor said that almost everyone in ICU ends up with it because it is so cold in there.

I thought, just great, his lungs were already in bad enough shape. He also said that Harry would take longer to heal because of the immunosuppressant drugs that he took. I never paid any attention to those statements because Harry had always healed quickly and this time was no exception.

Another day when I got there, I saw that they had cut his hair and shaved off his beard; he had a ponytail at the time. I told them that nobody had asked my permission to do this and they said they didn't want to bother with it. He looked so weak and sick like that, and I knew he would hate it if he knew.

Later on, he would tell me that he knew someone was shaving his face because they did it with a dry razor and he could feel the pain. He could hear a woman muttering, "they weren't going to bother with this hair no more."

This same moron had taken the respirator out of his mouth while she was cutting his hair and shaving his face and he heard her being told that people in critical condition could not have their respirators taken out for any reason. Harry heard her say, "big deal he gonna die anyway." I wonder how long it was out of his mouth before someone saw this idiot. She could have killed him.

After four weeks, Harry

finally started to improve and the doctors could not believe it. Harry was finally taken off the respirator, and slowly brought out of the coma. We had waited so long to hear his voice and when we did, it was total nonsense. He thought a cart rolling down the hall was a lion. He thought the people on the TV could see him. I was so upset; I thought he had brain damage. I was told it was just the effects of the drugs and the coma wearing off.

A couple of days later My Dad and I went to see Harry. His sister JoAnn had also come to visit that day. Harry had been in ICU for five weeks now and he was going to be moved to a private room. We all followed his bed down the hall and JoAnn and I were both crying; we were so happy that he was out of ICU.

Harry seemed so confused to be in a regular room. I hated to leave him there alone, but it was late in the day now and Dad did not want to drive home in the dark. The nurse there told me he still had a long road ahead to recovery, but at the time I didn't understand that at all. No one told me that he still had internal injuries that needed to be healed. I thought it was just a matter of him getting his strength back and getting back on his feet.

When I came back the next day, Harry was still pretty much disoriented. He didn't know where he was and it was all very scary for him. The effects of the coma were still wearing off and he had lost five weeks of his life. He was just starting to realize that he had almost died. He still had drains in his side and his stomach that drained amylase, which is pancreatic fluid.

When the doctor came in, he told Harry that his whole body was bathed in blood during the surgery and that he nicked his pancreas. He told Harry that he would probably have to have a tube put in his pancreatic duct to heal it. We didn't understand any of the technical terms of this, just that he was still very sick. Harry was now going to be turned over to a general surgeon for this problem.

September came and it was Harry's fiftieth birthday. He was glad to be alive, but could still not get out of bed; he was so weak and wobbly on his feet. Finally a kidney doctor came in and found out they were giving Harry double doses of blood pressure medicine in ICU and they had not bothered to drop the dosage back down yet.

Yet another incident of their constant incompetence, no one pays any attention to what's going on with the patient. The doctor smiled and told Harry he had added something to the kidney transplant experience, almost like he was glad it had happened because it was a wonderful experiment.

Mike was there with me that day and started to cry, and it finally came out that Harry had written that note in ICU that had said, "just let me die." This was the first time I had heard of it, Mike had bore the burden of these words to himself to protect me. It was so heartbreaking!

Harry told him he thought he was in a war in his coma and Agent Orange was being sprayed in the room. He was trying to tell us to save ourselves and just leave him there to die. The sounds of the machines in the next cubicle made him think this was happening. Even in a coma, he was thinking of his family and trying to protect us. Harry had always said that he would give his life for his family. Poor Mike, he had thought at the time that his Dad was giving up, but at least then he understood what Harry had been trying to say.

I brought Joe with me one night to see Harry, and I wanted to leave so that Joe could go to a school party. Harry was mad at us because we wanted to leave; and didn't understand why a party was more important than he was. I on the other hand didn't want the kid's lives to be any worse than they already were. This was Joe's senior year and I wanted to keep it at least semi-normal.

Harry came home on September 9, 2001. The reality of what had happened had finally set in, and we were very depressed. He was on a low protein diet to try and help heal his pancreas. The pancreas produces enzymes that help in the digestion of food and Harry had a hole in his, called a fistula.

He was still very ill; he had a JP drain in his side, short for Jackson Pratt that drained the pancreatic fluid into a small plastic bulb with a top that flipped open. This had to be constantly emptied and measured, the idea being that when the drain slowed down the pancreas was healed. He had another drain in his chest that was draining infection. We never knew it at the time, but it wasn't going to heal itself, it needed help. Harry walked around stooped over like an old man.

Two days after he was home, it was September 11, 2001. We heard about the twin towers in New York on the news and were scared and horrified. Shortly after we heard they had suspended air travel, we heard a plane go over our house. We just looked at each other and said, "who cares if we die." We had been through so much we just felt numb.

At our first visit to the general surgeon, he came in with a nasty frown on his face, looked at Harry and said, "Why didn't you let me do the surgery?" Could the man not read a medical chart? Harry did not choose anybody; he was life flighted in and a vascular surgeon was called. This doctor didn't want Harry for a patient if he wasn't the one who operated on him.

Harry and I said something

about what the vascular surgeon had told us about putting in a tube to drain the pancreas, and he totally ignored us. He was going to do what he wanted, which turned out to be nothing helpful that would end up healing Harry's pancreas. We stupidly let him do what he thought was best.

Harry needed home health care and a nurse would come to our house twice a week to take blood for tests, change his bandages and clean the area around his drains. She also took a sample of the fluid in his drain, and it was sent in to be tested for the amount of amylase in it. We literally lived to see the result of this test, but the numbers just stayed the same or sometimes were higher. He just never seemed to be getting any better and we were so depressed.

Harry told me while he was was in the coma in ICU, there was only one person that would come by and hold his hand and tell him he would be alright. He said he thought it was an angel because she was the only one to wear white. I told him that it was me because I always had on a white sweater. We both cried over that story.

CHAPTER SIX

The months went by and the drains in Harry never slowed down, the slightest movement would make the hole in his side bleed and run through the drain. The first time we saw blood in the drain, we were scared and thought he was bleeding internally. We called the on call doctors at night, and they as usual, had no idea why this was happening. Mike stayed up all night with Harry worrying. Later on, we found out that the tube inside him would irritate his skin and cause it to bleed and come out in the tube.

Another month went by and a dark brown fluid started coming out of the drain in Harry's side. Harry thought he had an infection.

161

The idiot doctor said it was that color because he had a kidney transplant. Come on, how stupid can you be? The doctors at the clinic literally know nothing about any other parts of the body except for their "so called specialty." And most of them refuse to consult with the other doctors there. So much for their famous "teamwork."

This doctor told us next to nothing about what was going on with Harry. Later we would understand that he just did not know what to do, and refused to ask anyone else for help. He would shake your hand with the tip of his fingers so that no one would crush his surgical fingers. And would then spend your ten-minute office visit staring at his expensive leather shoes and telling us nothing constructive.

Finally, when Harry came down with a fever, the doctor believed him and sent him to the infectious disease department. He had a staph infection and it was encapsulated in one area near the drain. This doctor kept telling Harry how serious it was and he didn't know if he could clear it up with antibiotics.

First, they tried pills that had no effect and then Harry had to have an IV tube put in his neck for antibiotics. He was on the strongest dose they had. The infectious doctor said this was a very, very serious infection and it would never clear up by itself. He was constantly saying that they would have to do surgery again to drain the infection out of there.

We were afraid that if they operated that the infection would spread and kill him. This doctor wasn't even a surgeon and no one else had suggested doing this. It was just another random opinion to scare us to death.

Harry ended up being on this antibiotic for months and was told that no one had ever been on this medicine for that long a time. The doctor wanted him to stop taking the medicine but we literally "willed" them not to. It was really strange because the doctor just sat there debating and we just kept thinking in our heads "don't do it, don't do it," and he suddenly said, "I won't do it." We just looked at each other in amazement.

What he didn't say was what we found out later; Harry had MRSA and the antibiotics could have caused a flesh eating disease if you were on them too long. So no matter what we wished, they were not doing what was best for the patient. We were just blessed that it turned out to be the right thing for Harry. We were glad we didn't know or we would have had to make a decision whether to stay on them or not.

We sat at home and just questioned everything in our life that led us to this moment. We had long ago thrown away our Catholic religion; however, there was still the brainwashed conviction from that religion that would come to mind; that we were being punished for something we did.

It is extremely difficult to try to wipe the religious slate clean and start over, especially when there is nothing to start over with. It is like being a man without a country. We had to sort through all of our emotions and beliefs and try to find some kind of faith.

One good thing that came out of this was that in almost losing each other, Harry and I became very close again. He told me that when he was on the helicopter that night going to Cleveland that he figured he was going to die and thought that this would not be a bad way to go. He would just close his eyes and that would be it. Then he remembered that he didn't get to say goodbye to the kids, so he had to live. And later, he saw his life being saved as a way to make up to the kids for the way he had treated them, and to make everything right. He never meant to hurt his sons.

Actually, when Harry came home it became even more stressful. When he was in the hospital, I had only myself and my feelings to deal with. Then I had to deal with Harry's feelings and how he felt about everything. I just cried constantly because it seemed like he was never going to get well.

Four months went by and it was almost Christmas. It seemed like nothing had changed much in Harry's condition. He had more energy but his pancreas still had not healed. The idiot doctor then decided to put Harry on TPN, which is Total Parental Nutrition. He sent Harry to another department to set this up. He was to have no food, no water, and was not even allowed to brush his teeth. This was supposed to help the pancreas heal, and it wouldn't have to work so hard if it didn't have to digest food.

TPN works by connecting two-liter fluid bags through an artery in your neck. The bags contained nutrition with sugar, amino acids, and electrolytes and a fat or lipid bag once a week. You need constant blood work to make sure that your nutrients are balanced. Harry was going to start this after the first of the year.

Right before Christmas, the medical supply truck pulled up with the bags of fluid and all the other supplies needed for TPN. Christmas and New Years was like having your last meal. It just got worse and worse with no end in sight.

At first, it was not so bad for Harry. He could even tolerate the sight of us eating as long as he didn't sit at the table with us. After a couple of weeks, he could not stand the smell of food. He would go down in the garage when we ate our meals. As time went on, we couldn't cook anything either; we all ate outside the house. It was so terrible for Harry; I don't know how he could stand it.

He kept saying that he always was ending up in the situation in life where there was no food to eat. Sometimes as a child, they didn't have much to eat, then during dialysis, when we lived in Denver and now this. This last experience has had a lasting effect on him.

Three months later, Harry was still on TPN. The lipid bag made him nauseous, lethargic, and his mouth was dry as dust. Liquid went into his neck via an infusion pump and there were problems with that sometimes. Alarms would go off if there was a malfunction in the machine and we would have to call the TPN people in the middle of the night to help reset the machine. He had to sleep on one side with a chair next to the bed to hold the machine. He would spend most nights sleeping in a recliner chair because it was more comfortable.

We started looking for someone else to help him. We finally made an appointment with a doctor in town who ended up sending us back to the clinic to see a college friend of his. The local doctor did not want to be involved in the mess the Cleveland Clinic had Harry in.

The general surgeon at the Cleveland Clinic found out we had an appointment with the gastrology department and cancelled the appointment. He was mad as hell and said we didn't need the other doctor. Against his wishes, Harry and I went ahead with it anyway.

The gastrologist wanted to put a stent in Harry's pancreas, which would bypass the fluid in the pancreas so that it could heal. We then understood that this is what the first vascular surgeon wanted to do. A tube was put down Harry's throat and the stent was inserted; it was to stay in there for two months.

After another month, Harry was getting really sick from the TPN. His glucose level was very high and he had to start giving himself insulin shots. When you are taking steroid drugs like Harry was for kidney rejection and you also have an infection, your body cannot process the large amounts of sugar. We learned about this afterwards, but the doctor was not smart enough to know it.

Instead, the idiot wanted Harry to stay on TPN indefinitely. That was it and Harry was worn down and had enough crap. He was afraid he would become diabetic next and it would harm his kidney transplant. It was not healing his pancreas anyway; we had more hope for the stent.

Both the TPN people and the gastrologist doctor asked the general surgeon what he had planned for Harry because he was not healing and the TPN was not working. The TPN people said they had never had a patient who was not allowed to swallow anything or even chew some gum. The general surgeon told them he was a doctor and he didn't need their opinions.

The end result was that Harry said he was taking himself off TPN, and everyone but the general surgeon agreed. He slowly started drinking fluids and eased himself back into solid food. This made him much healthier and able to heal easier.

The stent was finally taken out in April of 2002, but the tube was left in his neck for taking blood. It was still unclear whether his pancreas was healed because the abscess was covering the pancreas near the part where the fistula was. He still had the JP drain in his side, but the general surgeon decides to take that out and put in a long red tube. This tube would drain brown fluid constantly and ooze liquid around the tube soaking his clothes. One day, ten surgical staples poured out of his side along with the fluid.

Once when Harry was having a cat scan done, the technician took the tube out of his side for the test. When the procedure was over, the technician dropped the tube on the floor and before Harry could even blink, had put it back in his side. Harry was mad and told him he had not even sterilized the tube after he dropped it. The guy just said, "well, you're on antibiotics anyway, so it probably won't even matter."

He walked away and Harry demanded to know his name, but the other employees in the room would not tell him. This is the kind of people who work in radiology there. It's no wonder the Cleveland Clinic has such a high infection rate. He could have picked up countless other infections that the antibiotic would not cure and that would have compromised his health even more.

In June of 2001, Joe

graduated from high school. My Mom and Dad came and we all sat there together. I had tears in my eyes for more than one reason. Joe was our youngest son graduating and Harry was alive to be there to see it. We had Joe's graduation party two weeks later. Amy and Bill came home and helped us decorate the hall.

The day of the party, Harry was having trouble with the drain in his side and we thought both of us were going to miss the party. I just felt cheated out of everything in

life that day. We could not even enjoy a happy occasion. The drain cleared up in time for Harry to be there. My cousins helped us out that day. My Dad cooked and served the food. It was ninety-five degrees that day and I was so tired from being worried.

Two months later, my Mom called and told us that my Dad had just found out that he had pulmonary fibrosis, a disease of the lungs that causes scarring and shortness of breath. He was on oxygen and was going downhill fast. He was told he wouldn't live much longer. He couldn't do much for himself anymore and was very depressed. It was a horrible time for our whole family.

Later that month, Harry's doctor decides that the drain in his stomach can be removed. He didn't even take a cat scan to see if the infection in there had cleared up. Within twenty-four hours, Harry was really sick again and had a fever of 104. I knew that he would have to go back to the hospital. Harry told me "just let me die, I'm not going back to that place again. I can't take anymore." But we both knew he had to go, so I called the doctor's office and they told us to come to the clinic and he would be admitted.

It was five o'clock p.m. when we got there and we had to sit in the lobby four hours to wait for a room. Wouldn't you think the doctor could have arranged for a room before we got there? They don't care, sit in the lobby and suffer.

When he was finally admitted, they took him for a cat scan and saw that the drain which the incompetent moron had just removed was sitting dead center in the middle of the abscess, and that was the only way the infection had been draining out. I could have taken my bare hands and strangled that horrible doctor. His stupid incompetence had just about killed Harry. He had to have another JP drain put back in. I went home that night falsely thinking Harry would be alright at least until tomorrow.

The next morning before I got there, Harry called me and said his doctor had given orders for him to have a tube put down his throat for surgery. He had come in and told Harry that his pancreas was not healing and that the damaged part of it needed to be cut off. Harry asked him how he knew it wasn't healed and he just shrugged and said you can live without a part of it.

Well, that was it. Harry could not talk with the tube in his throat and when I got there, I called the ombudsman's office and told them I wanted another doctor. We had been considering this while Harry was still at home and I had the name of a doctor that we wanted to take over his case.

Once we found out that the doctor's do not work together there anyway, we knew we could get another. The ombudsman asked why I wanted this done, and I was yelling by then and told them I could write them a book by now about his lack of care and incompetence. He was removed from the case, and the tube was taken out of Harry's throat.

I went downstairs to get some lunch, and while I was gone, the fired doctor came to see him and he was furious. Harry asked him what his problem was, and the doctor told him "your wife is the problem." Harry wanted to tell him what he thought of him, but the doctor just walked away saying "I have real patients to see." Good riddance! At last, he was gone. The new doctor took over before Harry left the hospital.

In two weeks, Harry was home again and still on IV antibiotics. He was having cat scans done every two weeks to see if the abscess was receding. It was slowly shrinking down until one day the doctor could see that the pancreas was healed. He had the drain in his side removed, and Harry and I jumped for joy, it was the happiest day in a long time.

We also realized then that the first doctor was going to cut off a part of a perfectly good pancreas to cover up all his mistakes. Then no one would ever really know what had been wrong, and he probably would have killed Harry in the process. Things were really starting to look up after a year of misery.

It wasn't even a month later that more trouble came knocking at our door. I had not been to the gynecologist since before Harry had first been sick. People kept telling me I should go, but I ignored them. Finally, in August I was forced to go because I thought I had some kind of infection. My doctor took one look at me, and said I had abnormal white spots on my vulva and I would need to have a biopsy. For God's sake, what could happen next?

I had it done and when the results came back, the doctor called and wanted both of us to come in there and talk to her. I knew it was bad news then, I was scared to death.

I had second stage melanoma, and had to have surgery to have it removed. She said she was sending me to an oncologist specialist in cancer and she would do the surgery. I just sat there stunned, and Harry had tears in his eyes. We drove our car to a store parking lot and just sat there crying. We just could not take any more medical crisis; and now there was cancer to deal with and maybe even death.

We had not told the kids until we were sure of the results. When we got home, we sat down and talked to them. Mike looked as if someone had just taken his last breath away, and Joe just threw his head down on the table and cried. He could not stand something being wrong again.

Harry and I were both sick, and it was just the last straw. I guess that is when I really started to realize what Harry had felt. I was afraid when he was so sick that he would die, but I was never in the position to be the one who thought they were dying. I remember just looking out the window and wondering if I would be alive next summer. I had the time to think about my life and everything I would miss.

Harry also got to see things from my point of view, what it would be like if I was to die. Needless to say, we were just shocked. Harry blamed himself, thinking it was probably all the stress I had been under that had brought on the cancer. Actually it was probably true, but it wasn't his fault.

My Mother was beside herself; my Dad, Harry and I all had really serious medical problems. And she had barely recovered from the cancer she had a year ago herself. It just seemed like it was never going to end.

I was sent to an oncologist at one of the major hospitals. She told me the doctor in town was really smart to have noticed that those spots were cancer. If they had been left much longer, it would have been more serious. The surgery would consist of cutting off two inches of skin and sending them for a biopsy to make sure there was no more cancer.

The doctor decided that the other side of my vulva had a red look to it and that she also would cut off part of that skin in surgery and biopsy it. The surgery was scheduled for the first part of September.

The day of the surgery came and I had to be at the hospital at six in the morning to prepare for surgery. Harry, I, and the kids all went there together. Joe had a cold that day, and just slept in the chair most of the day. The surgery was delayed two hours because the person before me had complications. Everyone in the waiting room was getting worried.

Finally, five hours later, when the surgery was over, the doctor came out to talk to them, and said I was doing fine. Harry said he thinks she felt sorry for them, Joe was sick and Harry had his IV antibiotic bag rolling along with him, and the doctor just shook her head. What a mess we all were.

Nobody got to see me until ten o'clock that night. I stayed overnight in the hospital and then came home. I had stitches in me and had to lie on the couch for a month. I couldn't walk around except to go to the bathroom so that I wouldn't rip out the stitches. The kids were doing the wash, the dishes and everything, and by this time Harry was getting better and could help; he and Mike did my jobs at night.

My test results came back and thank God, there was no more cancer, it had all been removed in the original biopsy. I had the stitches taken out, and was numb for a year. But I was alive, and that was the important part.

Harry had his last drain taken out of him that fall, the infection was gone and his pancreas was healed. He was going to be able to go back to work in

December. We just had this wonderful feeling you have when you feel like you have beaten death. It was no doubt a miracle.

My Dad was glad for him, but he was getting sicker. I didn't have the time to pay attention to how sick my Dad was because of everything Harry and I were going through. And I later found out that Dad had pretended to be fine when he saw me because he knew I couldn't take anymore. That was his final gift to me, and I will love him always for it.

My sister Amy, her husband Bill and daughter Emily were coming home for Christmas because Dad was so sick. We all knew this would be our last Christmas together. Harry and I went over to Mom and Dad's to get their Christmas stuff out. My Dad was very upset that he couldn't help. He somehow got the strength to put up the Christmas tree, he so badly wanted to do it. He was trying to hold on until Christmas.

On December 16, my Dad had a heart attack caused by not having enough oxygen in his lungs. He fell to the floor in the bathroom and couldn't get back up. Mom called the rescue squad and told me while they were waiting that Dad was looking down the hall as if he saw someone. She thinks that someone was coming for him because he was dying. When the EMS came, they revived him and took him to the hospital. He didn't want to go because he said he would be ruining Christmas. Mom tried to tell him that he might be home in a few days.

They put him on a respirator until they could access his condition. My Mom and Dad had living wills that they were not to be kept alive by a breathing machine. My Mom didn't want him on the respirator and I told her at least let them see what the prognosis was. I was the only one in the room with my Dad when he opened his eyes. He looked at me and I could tell he looked panicked and I promised him we would not leave him like that for long.

I went all to pieces; it was the same scenario all over again as with Harry. A respirator and an induced coma. The doctors said his lungs were like stone, and there was no hope. I did not trust doctors by this point. My Mom thought she was going against his wishes keeping him on the respirator, but I could not make this decision. My sister, Amy came as fast as she could and arrived the next day and stayed with Mom that night. I felt physically ill watching another illness like this.

By morning, my Mom and Amy had decided that we should let Dad go. He was always there for me, so how could I help decide to let him die? Mom and Amy talked to me and in the end; I could not let him suffer like that either.

I came back to the hospital and they took him off the

respirator. They kept him in the coma so he wouldn't be uncomfortable. His lungs gave out in a half hour and then his heart. I had never seen anyone die before, but on that day, I believed in life after death. Within seconds, you could tell it was not my Dad anymore, his body was an empty shell, and his spirit was gone.

Everyone came back to Mom's. Bill and Emily had come from Florida that morning, and Harry, Mike and Joe came from work. Harry had only been back to work for three days. Joe was so upset he couldn't stand anymore.

So, since it was so close to Christmas, we had the funeral within three days. I didn't even have any tears left to shed, so much had happened. This seems to be a bad time of year for our family. My great grandmother, grandmother, grandfather, Uncle, and cousin all died in December right before Christmas, and now my

Dad.

It was odd, but is seemed that my Dad's death was the very thing that brought Amy and I together. We had never been close, but we have been from that day on. Amy stayed with Mom through the New Year and then she had to go back home. Mom then had to start her life over alone.

In January of that next year, Mike called us one night and said his car had skidded on the ice and his truck was totaled. Harry and I went to the site of the accident and could not believe that Mike was just standing there. His truck had gone off the road, went through an entire grove of trees, and never harmed him. By the looks of that truck, we knew we had been blessed again. Our son was alright!

The year of 2003 was a good year. We had been through sickness and death and felt that wonderful calmness that comes when you have been through hell and have come out in one piece on the other side. We knew without a doubt that a miracle had happened. We were shocked and in awe. We were both alive and healthy, but my Dad was gone. Harry and I were closer than we had been in years.

Early in the year, I was in the emergency room in our hometown with a sinus infection and came across the doctor that had been there the night Harry had almost died. I thanked him for his quick thinking, which had contributed to saving Harry's life.

He told me "you will probably think I am crazy, but when I saw your husband come in that night, God spoke to me. He told me that this is a seriously ill man, and I need to do something right away." I told him that I absolutely believed him because everything that had happened that night was part of the miracle that saved Harry's life. It is the most awe-inspiring feeling to have had a part in a miracle.

CHAPTER SEVEN

That winter Harry had connected online with some old friends that he had as neighbors in Ripley. They started talking about a house on their street that was listed in a book called "Haunted Ohio."

There was also a house next to the one Harry lived in that had been owned by an old woman. They told Harry that no one had been able to rent it and they couldn't sell it because one of the rooms was ice cold all the time and the bedroom door wouldn't stay open. That was a spooky street. Of course, that led to telling the story of the grapes on the wallpaper that would swish back and forth.

Harry's friend told him that the house that they had lived in on the same street was haunted also. They had a big old house with a bathroom off every bedroom and a fireplace in each room. This girl and her sister would lie in bed at night and see some old man that was ghostlike sitting in the bathtub taking a bath. Other things happened in their house like people walking down the steps when no one was there. The whole block was haunted, and I thought this was very interesting.

We went to Ripley that summer because one of Harry's childhood friends was coming to visit from Florida. We visited with her, and old neighbors and friends. Harry had not seen any of these people in thirty years, so there was a lot of catching up to do. I felt right at home there. They just accepted me as one of the family, since they felt that way about Harry.

While we were there, we found

out that Harry's Aunt Nancy and her husband were living right across the street. We went and saw her, and she was just like I thought she would be. Here was a person who had cared about her first husband, and had good stories to tell about Harry's Dad and his brothers. She told us about going hunting with Harry's grandpa, and how living in the old Greiner house up on the hill was like going camping.

Nancy and her second husband had lived on a farm on the outskirts of town for years. She told us Bob and Hilda used to come out and visit with them and bring Harry and his sisters. After Nancy's mother died, they moved back into her house in town. Nancy was born there and was happy to come home. I could feel the history in the house the minute I walked in there.

She took us upstairs and showed us the room that her first husband, Herman, had died in. She told us Herman had constant nosebleeds and had high blood pressure, and was turned down for the military because of this. Finally, he was so sick that he went to the doctor. The doctor took a urine sample, and it was boiled in a type of Bunsen burner, and the albium in it was so thick and white that the doctor said it was malignant; his kidneys were failing. It was 1946, and little was known about kidney disease.

Nancy was told to take him home and put him to bed, so she took him to her mother's house in town. Herman asked Nancy if she would have married him if she had known that this would happen. Her answer to him will remain personal, but I know it would have been yes because she loved him. She said she lost twenty pounds in the two weeks before he died, and being so young, could not understand him dying like he did.

Nancy said that Ollie Belle, who was Harry's grandmother, had died because of a problem with her kidneys. That was all they knew in 1933. Herman had been afraid that he had the same problem as his mother. That was more horrible than I even imagined. I had always known somewhere inside me that Nancy would have loved him and this story broke my heart.

I went back to the hotel after that and cried. I hid my tears from Harry because it upset him when I let this stuff get to me. Those stories just always struck a chord in my heart. It was ridiculous, but it always felt like I was there when it happened because I could envision it so clearly.

The fear of this disease has lived through the generations, first Ollie, then Herman, Bob, Harry and my fear for my children. It was a nightmare to know ahead of time that this might happen. But at least our generation did not fear death.

That trip was a time for

stories. Phyllis, who had been a good friend of Hilda's, was telling us the story of Hilda finding out that Bob and then Harry had kidney disease. She told us she remembered when Harry's Dad got sick and it was so horrible and that there was no money and no hope for him.

Eight years after that, Phyllis was with Hilda when she got the news that Harry also had kidney disease. After Harry had the kidney biopsy, the hospital called with the bad news. She said Hilda just dropped to the floor and sobbed, "Not my son, not my son too." I can feel her sorrow, and it breaks my heart to think of it.

We came back home and I filed all this information away in my head. Writing this book was nagging at me, almost like the Greiner's that had gone before wanted me to write it. I just could not get these people out of my mind. The rest of the summer and fall were peaceful.

In January of the next year 2004, Joe went on a vacation to Colorado where he was born. All of his friends were sick with some virus while they were there, and he said he was sick too. He was not due to come home for several days and I was worried because he was so far away from home.

Meanwhile, Harry started having bad pains that would double him over like bad indigestion. They would come and go. This went on for several days. I wanted him to see a doctor, but he kept thinking they would go away. We were all paranoid as far as seeing doctors by then.

When Joe came home, he was sicker than I had ever seen him because he had not seen a doctor there. He had an ear and sinus infection. He had to see our doctor immediately. He was on an antibiotic and had to stay home from work.

Harry pains were getting worse, and one night it was so bad I told him that we should go to the ER and have him checked out. I was a nervous wreck; I was afraid of what was wrong with him and the ER was nothing but bad memories for me.

They took a bunch of tests and said his pancreas was acting up. I was just so mad and scared; I just kept saying that I knew it was too good to be true that we thought he was healed. I refused to talk to anyone, I was so upset. He was admitted to the hospital and I went home to be with Joe because he was so sick.

The next day I went back to the hospital and the doctor came in and said that Harry was having gallbladder attacks. He would have to have surgery to remove his gallbladder. The CAT scan showed a strange mark on his pancreas, and since he had all those problems with it at the Cleveland Clinic, they suggested he go back there to have the CAT scan looked at. The doctors at the clinic refused to talk to the doctors here, so we had no choice but to go back there.

The attacks calmed down and Harry was well enough to go home, and we had to make an appointment in Cleveland. We saw the doctor who had taken over his case during the aneurysm. He said the mark on his pancreas was scar tissue from the fistula he had in there during the aneurysm.

We went home and the surgery was scheduled to be done in two weeks. It was going to be done laproscopically if possible and the recovery would be quick.

Mike and I went there the day of the surgery, Joe was still sick and taking his second set of antibiotics. We waited in the same crappy waiting room you always have to wait in. The surgery was to take two hours, and four hours later we were so worried that Mike had to go up to the desk to ask what was going on.

Well of course, they had to do the open surgery because there was too much scar tissue in his stomach to do it laproscopically. So now, Harry had a double set of scars from this surgery. He remarked later that we could just call him Frankenstein because he had so many scars from all of his surgeries.

He came out of the surgery alright and would have to be in the hospital about a week. I asked the surgeon how his kidney function was and he just gave me a dirty look and was totally insulted. I didn't think it was an odd question, but I guess you don't question anyone's surgical ability at the Cleveland Clinic. Well, I did

One day our nephew Jon and his wife were going to the clinic so that Jon could be tested to get on the kidney transplant list. I rode along with them to see Harry. That day stands out so vividly in my mind.

We came out of the parking garage and I was going one way into the main part of the hospital and Jon was going the other way into the clinic part of the hospital where the doctors were. I looked at his face and he seemed so young that I had tears in my eyes when he walked away. I could imagine it being my own son going to that appointment.

After that day, I never got back to visit Harry again. I ended up with the virus Joe had, I was sick, and I still had to work at night. Joe had not wanted us to worry about him with everything else going on, but the antibiotic he was taking was not agreeing with him, in fact it was making him sicker; his vomit was green and he had severe diarrhea.

Mike and I took Joe to the emergency room and waited half the night to get things straightened out. I think Mike and I were beside ourselves. I just sat there so sick and Mike just kept ranting about how Joe should have told us he was so sick, and then we wouldn't be there.

I tried to ignore him until I finally had to tell Mike to shut up, that no matter what, Joe was ours and we were going to take care of him. Mike later apologized to me and said he was just so upset. We had all had it with hospitals.

Meanwhile, Harry was at the Cleveland Clinic, and his roommate was a minister. This man had been through some very serious surgery and the doctors and nurses there were giving him no encouragement to get well as usual. Harry told him his story of nearly dying and tried to encourage him to believe he would get well in spite of what they said there. It started to work and the minister got better every day. They really work hard to lower your morale there.

This minister would lie in bed and listen to his sermons on a cassette player. One day, a male nurse from Iraq came in and started giving his unsolicited opinion to Harry and the minister. He asked them if they believed in this Jesus person with the Virgin Mother and was scoffing at the idea. He told them the United States should stay in their own backyard and out of their business in Iraq.

Harry reported him to a staff doctor and they said there was nothing they could do about him. One of the nurses said this guy was like that in nursing school, but no one there did anything about him either. Harry and the minister were afraid to sleep at night when he was there. Harassment in a hospital bed, but that was nothing unusual for Harry; it had happened to him before at the Cleveland Clinic.

By the time Harry was ready to go home, Joe and I were finally well. Carol and I went to pick up Harry at the hospital. Within a month, he was healed and everything was back to normal.

Joe was working at a drug store about 25 miles from home. He had been transferred there from Norwalk and had a good job with benefits. He was always tired; he would fall asleep all the time. I tried to convince myself that it was his hectic life, but it reminded me of the stories of Harry when he was in end stage renal failure.

That spring Mike moved into his own apartment. He had wanted to move a couple years earlier, but he stayed because Harry was so sick. We were sad to see him go, but it was good to see him on his own. We helped Mike settle into his new place, and everybody was happy.

We spent the rest of the year doing normal things, and were moving on with our lives. We were sure all the bad times were over. After all, what could happen worse than Harry nearly dying?

In the spring of 2005, Joe started having problems at work, and was becoming very upset. This went on for weeks and his blood pressure was slightly high. This scared me, but it was our turn for denial, and we brushed it off because he was so upset. He was alright otherwise and things seemed to calm down after awhile.

That summer we went to Ripley again. Harry's childhood friend, David Gast, lived in a nearby town and he wanted to come to Ripley and see Harry. They had a good reunion; they hadn't seen each other since 1976 when we were in Ripley and stayed with him and his wife. We all piled into his van and took a ride through the country so they could reminisce about the past.

He drove us up to the house the Greiner's had lived in for a hundred years, since we couldn't remember how to get there again. We got out and knocked on the door, but no one was home. I would love to see the inside of that house someday.

We visited some neighbors and Harry's Aunt Nancy. We went to the graveyard and took pictures of the gravestones of Harry's ancestors for my genealogy research. We stayed a couple of days and went home. It was a strange and kind of melancholy trip.

When we came back from Ripley, Joe asked me if Harry had any living relatives, and the age-old question came up of what had happened to them. I told him they had died of kidney disease. He told me he was going to be really pissed off if he ever got that disease.

About a month later, we realized that Joe's blood pressure was getting higher. Again, we do nothing and are in denial until it is really high. It was then I knew why Hilda waited so long to see a doctor when Harry got sick.

I called Harry at work and

told him I was taking Joe to the ER. There was no sense going to the doctor and waiting for the results of a million tests. I knew the answer anyway and the waiting would kill me. Harry met me at the hospital.

So here it was, again August 8, the same day I found out I had cancer and the same day Harry had the aneurysm surgery. Needless to say, I would hate that date from that day on. Harry was still hoping it was something else, but I knew better. I was a mess and Harry made me wait in the waiting room so I wouldn't upset Joe.

I just paced up and down the hall crying because I knew he was going to come out and tell me that Joe had kidney disease, my worst nightmare. I selfishly was glad he made me wait outside, because I could not stand to see Joe's face when they told him. I had seen enough of that the night they told Harry he would probably die.

They did several tests and

finally realized from something that Joe said that our family had kidney disease. I myself would have told them to check that first, but I wasn't there. Harry came out and told me they were checking his urine. I knew this was it. When Harry came back out again, he said they had told Joe his kidneys weren't working well, and they were admitting him to the hospital.

John and Carol called Joe; they both understood what we were going through. Dee Dee, my lifelong friend, and her daughter Amber came to visit that day. I had to go to work, so I went home for awhile. I got home and just screamed "NO, NO, NO!" to the empty house. Even though I knew, I just could not believe that what I had always feared had finally happened. It was just too painful.

The nephologist came in the next day and we told him about the family having glomulernephritis, and he asked what kind. Well for all the years we refused to even discuss the subject, we didn't know. How stupid could we be? Anyway, we needed to find out or they were going to do a kidney biopsy.

I called Harry's doctor in Cleveland and found out it was called FSGS. Familiar focal segmented glomerical sclerosis. I had never even heard the word until then. Since we knew what it was, they didn't do a biopsy; his blood pressure was too high anyway to have this procedure done. Joe had to stay in the hospital until it went down. He was on large doses of blood pressure pills with all kinds of weird side effects, and he was scared and very angry and unhappy.

The nephrologist at the hospital said Joe should have a fistula put in his arm because he would probably be on dialysis by November. Joe's creatinine, the test to measure kidney function was already 4.7. I could not believe this had all happened so fast and that he was already in end stage renal failure. We put off the fistula for awhile, we had to think and we didn't trust doctors or their opinions. I later wished we had listened and had it done then. The misery we could have saved Joe!

About a week later, Joe's blood pressure was down and he went home. We were all severely depressed. We just kept telling Joe how sorry we were, but words were not enough. Harry and I blamed ourselves; we should never have had any children. Harry said he was worthless and just bred disease and I said that I knew better and I had children anyway.

We could have helped Joe cope with this better if we had not been such a wreck ourselves. Because no matter what, it had happened and he would have to find some way to deal with it.

This just brought up all the bad things that had ever happened to Harry in his life. I had often told him to think of some pleasant memory from his childhood. He said he could not remember any. He was always like a man without a past.

In our grief, we made our first mistake. Harry's doctor in Cleveland said he would see Joe. We had to get him in to see a doctor and this was no time to start searching for anew place to go. We mistakenly thought that the kidney department at the Cleveland Clinic was alright and we were familiar with the people there.

We took Joe to Cleveland at the end of August 2005. The doctor offered us a new treatment that would prevent the disease from advancing so quickly. We stupidly thought this might work and give us all some time to adjust to all this, and prevent dialysis by finding a donor in time.

Joe was going to be given cellcept, an immunosuppressant drug that would help slow down the progression of kidney disease. And he also needed to have a kidney biopsy to determine how far the disease had progressed.

In September, Joe had the kidney biopsy and had to stay overnight in the hospital because you have to lay flat on your back for several hours after the procedure so you don't bleed to death.

Several days later after he was back home, the doctor called with the results. Joe definitely had FSGS. We stupidly hoped against hoped that the answer might be different.

We had a lot of people praying for Joe, I even prayed to Harry's and my father in heaven, but to no avail. I guess some things are just inevitable. Harry and I just could not bear the pain of what was happening.

Harry was thankful that he could be there for Joe to help him, as his own father could not be there for him. The rest of

Harry's family just acted like it was something normal, and that irritated me to no end. Carol felt a little differently because her son Jon was also on dialysis.

Joe started on the drugs to delay kidney disease and it was a nightmare we should have avoided. He kept having bladder spasms from the pills. They changed the pills twice and they had the same effect. The day of his 22nd birthday, he was having terrible spasms. He could not even have one normal day.

Joe was still trying to work during this time. I remember him coming home one day with the bladder spasms, and he was so mad he punched his hand onto the living room floor and broke his wrist. Therefore, we spent another day in the emergency room.

He had a cast on his arm with everything else going on and he was all doped up with pain pills that night. The pills to delay kidney disease didn't work and were a waste of time; they only caused more trouble. But we were grasping at straws and were willing to try anything.

Well, it didn't work and the next step was dialysis. Harry remembered how awful hemodialysis was; having a tube put in your arm and being connected up to a machine and being so sick. So we chose peritoneal dialysis. Nancy and Norma were on this and it could be done at home.

We were sent to a center in Cleveland, not far from the clinic for instructions. There were two ways to do this. You could be on a machine while you slept at night or do hand exchanges four times a day. The machine would put fluid in your peritoneal cavity in your stomach, drain it back out several times a night, and clean the poisons out. In the hand exchanges, you drained a bag of fluid into your stomach and then connected another bag to drain the poisons back out with the fluid.

Either way, in order to do this you had to have a tube put in your peritoneal cavity through your stomach during a surgical procedure. A more improved procedure than when Harry had it done, but the method was still the same. Joe had this done in October; he was admitted to the hospital and had the surgery to put the tube in his stomach for dialysis. He stayed overnight again and went home the next day. It was very uncomfortable having the tube in there and you had to be very careful of infection.

We were driving to Cleveland once a week for the dialysis classes. Joe was depressed but was taking all this in his stride at the time. The head of nephrology from the Cleveland Clinic would see the patients at this center once a week. He wanted Joe to be in a movie about young renal patients that exercise while on dialysis. We just thought, "who the hell wants to do this?" This is not a happy time and they just wanted to use him for publicity for the Cleveland Clinic. We said no.

Meanwhile, we had four people offer to donate a kidney to Joe. Myself, Harry's sister Chris, and two women who were friends of ours. They would not put Joe on the transplant list until his creatinine reached a certain level. I later found out that other transplant centers don't do this. They try to line up donors right away to avoid dialysis. The clinic just drags everything out. The patient is in better health and better spirits if dialysis can be avoided.

We had to go to a couple of meetings to meet with transplant coordinators so they could explain dialysis and the steps that you would have to take until you have a transplant. Joe also met with one of the living donor transplant coordinators, and saw a transplant surgeon. He also had to see a psychologist to make sure he was in the right frame of mind and that he would be capable of taking care of himself and his transplant.

The donors all had to be spoken to and tested. The living donor transplant coordinator only worked part time and was impossible to get on the phone. The donors were all complaining to us that the clinic just didn't seem very interested in them donating a kidney.

These people spent a lot of their time making phone calls trying to give Joe a kidney. We thought at the time that this was really a poor way to run a kidney transplant program. The clinic didn't seem to care about this program anymore now that heart transplants were the current thing for them to boast about.

I was a good match for Joe, but was turned down because of the cancer I had a couple of years before. They said I might have a stray cancer cell in my kidneys.

Another person was turned down because of some medication that they were taking. It came down to Chris and one other woman. They both had to lose weight to be a donor.

Other people offered but gave up trying when no one would answer or return any of their calls at the clinic. They told us that this gave them a bad feeling and they had heard about so many negative outcomes at the clinic. They said they were sorry, but they didn't feel right about donating anymore because they didn't feel that they could trust them.

The first day that Joe was on dialysis in Cleveland, they did a hand exchange. It was November 11, and all of our lives we had constantly seen 11:11 on our clock. We had always questioned what that could mean, and on that day we knew we had the answer.

That same day, while we were there, Chris called us on her cell phone and said she was accepted to be the donor. We were so excited. We thought the surgery would be soon and Joe would not have to be on dialysis for long. We were so grateful to Chris for offering; she was after all a family member.

We had all decided that Joe would be on the peritoneal dialysis machine that would run during the night. We took the machine home with us that day and set it up in Joe's room. It just made me sick to look at it there. It was sitting in the same spot where I had seen it in my vision years ago.

The medicine truck was coming to our house again but this time it was delivering supplies and bags of dialysis fluid. Oh how I hated to see that truck come to our door again. It reminded me of all those TPN bags when Harry was sick. It just seemed like our family was forever in some kind of medical crisis.

Joe went to a hockey game that night with a friend, saying he was

not going to be able to do
anything at night anymore because
he had to be on dialysis by nine
at night in order to be able to go
to work in the morning. We felt so
bad for him, twenty-two years old
and stuck with this life. The
first doctor in our hometown had
been right; he was on dialysis by
November.

The first night he was hooked
up to the machine, it went well
for the first hour or so. When it
came to the cycle to drain the
fluid out of him, he was in
extreme pain and he couldn't stand
the pressure in his stomach. He
kept yelling to stop the machine.
We had to let the fluid drain out
and then we stopped the machine.
It was a horrible sight to watch
and I was scared to death about
what would happen. We knew then we
would have to do the hand
exchanges.

We started them the next
morning. Most people did three
exchanges during the day and the

last one at ten at night, that way you could sleep through the night. Since Joe worked during the day, we had to do one in the morning, one after work, the next one at ten at night, and the last one at two in the morning. That way the long period could be during the day instead of at night.

We were all so tired, and had to be alert in the middle of the night. Harry did the dialysis treatments, I was too nervous I would do something wrong. We had to wear masks and be very careful about cleanliness to avoid infection. There is a high risk of peritonitis, which is an infection in your peritoneal cavity in your stomach, if germs touch any of the tubes.

We had to go to the dialysis center once a week for blood tests and to see the doctor. They had to make sure that the dialysis was cleaning the poisons out of Joe's body properly. One good thing about this dialysis was that you could drink everything you wanted and eat a few more foods than you could on hemodialysis.

The bad thing was that his stomach would sometimes fill up with blood from the tube being irritated and you would have to do extra exchanges with very cold fluid to seal the area where the blood was leaking from until the blood was all filtered out. It was all so scary.

Meanwhile, the clinic was dragging their feet to have the donor tests done on Chris. There were not enough doctors to see the patients so it took months to set up the tests.

Chris's were set up to start in January of 2006. It just seemed to be taking forever to get them to move along so Joe could have his transplant. We saw no excuse for this, when you have a donor, they should proceed right away so the kidney patient is not so worn down by dialysis, and can get on with their new life. But the

Cleveland Clinic doesn't care about their patients or their feelings.

Also during this time, Joe was having trouble with his vision. He made an appointment with the eye doctor and he came home and told us the doctor thought he had an eye disease called keratoconus. The corneas is your eyes are odd shaped and sometimes if it gets bad enough you need to have a cornea transplant at some point. My sister Amy and my niece, Emily also have this. Joe was really upset, and said he must have come out on the bottom of the gene pool in our family.

We took Joe to see a specialist and they told him there was a good possibility that his eyes would not get any worse and that he needed to wear hard contacts. Our doctor tried over and over but could not get the contacts to fit. Joe was constantly going to doctors and everything seemed like a medical battle. We finally got Joe to another doctor who knew what she was doing. So that was finally straightened out.

Norma had gotten remarried and Thanksgiving was at her house that year. Hilda's health had declined and she had been put in a nursing home earlier in the year, and Nancy brought her for the day. Carol's kidney transplant was going bad after twenty years and the topic was dialysis and the menu for kidney patients.

How depressing! Carol was going to go on hemodialysis, and she and Joe were talking about that. Hilda just sat there in her wheelchair and offered no comment at all. I'm not sure if she understood, or just couldn't stand the subject.

Amy and her family came home for Christmas that year, so it wasn't as sad as it would have been. We consoled ourselves by saying that next year would be a happy one since Joe would have had his transplant by then.

The first of the year came and Chris started having her tests to donate her kidney. Harry went with her to all of her doctor's appointments. She had a cat scan done of her kidneys so they could decide which one to take. Then urine samples, a pap test, an angiogram of her kidney and tons of other tests to make sure she was healthy. She was told she would have to lose some weight in order to have laparoscopic surgery done.

After the tests were done she saw a nephrologist who said she was the most "disgustingly healthy person" he had seen in a long time. She was really happy about that since she so badly wanted to donate a kidney to Joe.

She also had to talk to a psychologist so they could be sure that she was emotionally stable to donate a kidney and that she was doing this of her own free will.

They want to make sure that someone is not being forced to donate and they are not doing it out of guilt. Joe had seen this same doctor.

Joe and Chris had blood tests taken every week to make sure that none of their antibodies changed before the transplant.

In March, Chris had her first appointment with her surgeon. Harry didn't like him the first time he saw him. But the doctors there tend to be arrogant, so that wasn't necessarily a sign that he was incompetent. She told him if for any reason they had to switch to an open surgery she was still willing to donate. The only thing that mattered to her was that Joe have a good kidney.

The surgeon was a cocky foreign doctor who told her not to worry, "he was the best in the world and could do this surgery in his sleep." He claimed that he had done thousands of them. She would later wish that he had been asleep; it might have turned out better.

He told her they had decided to take her left kidney, and put it in Joe's right side. She was never told the risks of this surgery in any of these appointments. He just kept bragging about how great he was. She was assured that everything would be fine.

Chris felt very confident that everything would turn out good for her and Joe. We were all concerned for Chris because she had never had surgery before, and we hoped it would not be too painful for her. This made her doubly courageous to volunteer for this.

The transplant was to be at the end of March. Two weeks before it was to take place, the clinic came up with the idea of using Chris and Joe's surgeries in the kidney symposium they were planning for April, which was kidney donation month.

They were going to film the surgery with the clinic transplant team, visiting surgeons and UNOS members as observers. We were told this would be used for publicity for publicity for kidney donation, and for educational purposes. There would also be a short story about it on the news channels in northeast Ohio the morning of the surgery.

The clinic told us Chris and Joe were the healthiest people on the transplant schedule, which made them the best candidates for the surgery that they wanted to film. They said they didn't expect any complications. Really, they just knew our family history and knew this would be a good background story for the big hoopla they were planning, but we didn't realize this at the time. We were hesitant to do this, but were assured that they would have the very best surgical team, the two top surgeons, and the best care since this was being filmed. The kidney transplant was scheduled for April 6, 2006.

After that the madness really started. I got calls from all kinds of people from different departments of the Cleveland Clinic asking me the family history of the Greiner's. The urologists, the nephrologists, the media department, they all asked the same endless questions over and over. What were the names of the Greiner's who had died of kidney disease? Where did the disease start in Harry's family? Did his dad die at the Cleveland Clinic? I told them he had died in Cincinnati. Were they even going to exploit his death?

It was all very upsetting, and we didn't need all those reminders of the past with Joe having the same disease. It was like a dark shadow over the whole new hope of Joe's transplant. They were digging up all this crap just for publicity for the Cleveland Clinic.

We all felt like we wanted to

back out of this media circus, but the date of the transplant was set and we wanted Joe to be well again. The clinic even contacted our local newspaper and they did a story on our family. We just really didn't want all this stress; we had enough as it was.

Joe and Chris went to the clinic a week before the transplant. The media department filmed Joe going up to the desk to check in, and then they took him into the exam room with the surgeon, lined up the cameras, and instructed him and Joe what to say. The surgeon was a nervous bumbling wreck. He had no clue what to say. He just explained what would happen next week during the transplant. Joe told him that people had said he had to be the best because he was the head of the transplant surgical team.

Joe hates now that he ever told him that. He and Chris were like two lambs going to the slaughterhouse. They trusted those two doctors. Nancy and Norma came with us that day because the media department wanted to do interviews with the family about Joe's transplant and their personal feelings about their own kidney transplants. Carol and John didn't want to be a part of it.

We were taken into the lobby of the international hotel in the clinic where we were all interviewed. These segments were going to be intertwined into the movie of the surgery. I hated the idea as I don't like to be in the spotlight, but I did it for Joe.

Harry cried because he still felt like the cause of all this. I said I hoped Joe would be like his Dad and still have his transplant thirty-four years later. Nancy and Norma were teary eyed.

Chris and Joe were simply heartbreaking in their stories of how they hoped the transplant would turn out. Joe in his desire for a new healthy life and Chris so badly wanting to help a member of the family. She had wanted to donate for Nancy and Norma when they needed a kidney, but she was too young at the time.

The media department told us that someone would most likely come to interview us from the TV station the day of the surgery. They asked us if we had any problems in the past with the Cleveland Clinic. Harry said oh yes we had! We were told that if we mentioned anything negative about the Cleveland Clinic then the surgery wouldn't take place. So we had to remain silent for Chris and Joe.

CHAPTER EIGHT

The next week, Chris, Joe, Harry and I came to the clinic the day before the transplant. Chris was hesitant that day about going. We should have taken that as an omen. We didn't pressure her and she finally decided that she would go. Chris and Joe had to have the final tests and blood work drawn before the transplant.

That night we had arranged to stay at the clinic inn across the street on the floor for transplant families. It was a dirty place run by foreigners, but we could not afford to stay at the expensive international hotel at $250.00 a night at that time.

Joe had his last dialysis treatment that night and we were so happy that we were done with that for good. We were all so nervous we barely slept that night. We had to be at the surgery center at five the next morning.

Morning came and Chris and Joe were taken and prepped for surgery. We sat with each of them until they were taken into surgery. They were both very nervous. Neither one of them were asked to sign a consent form for the surgery. This fact would not occur to us until much later on.

Nancy and Norma came to the clinic the day of the surgery and brought Mike with them. The media department came and said the news channels were not interested in an interview about the transplant. Kidney transplants were not top news anymore.

We were relieved; we didn't want to talk to anyone anyway. In fact, we had already decided we were done with this publicity circus. This day was about Joe, Chris, and the transplant, and that was our only concern that day. The woman with the media department was still talking about making some story out of this, but we couldn't have cared less.

After two hours, we got the call that Chris' part of the surgery was over and that she was alright. A couple of hours later, Nancy and Norma went to see Chris in recovery. Harry, Mike and I waited for news about Joe.

Two hours after that Harry was called to the telephone and the transplant surgeon said Joe was out of surgery and the transplant had worked. Harry said the doctor seemed very nervous. Neither one of these doctors came out to talk to any of us in person.

We got to see Joe in recovery several hours later. I hated seeing all those tubes and wires coming out of him. I knew he was alright, but it was an upsetting sight. I'm glad that I did not know then that he really wasn't alright.

Chris was put in a private room in the fancy part of the hospital that they reserve for transplant donors and celebrities. The room was nice, but that floor was not run any different than any other part of hospital. Chris was in a lot of pain, but she seemed to be alright. We felt bad for her because I don't think she knew how painful it would be.

Nancy was going to stay there overnight with Chris and take care of her. Carol, John and his wife and kids came to the clinic to see Chris. Joe didn't get back to a regular room until 11:30 that night, so no one got to see him. He was asleep most of the night anyway.

We had rented the room at the clinic inn until Joe could be released from the hospital. At first we both went back and forth to sleep at night, but we could tell Joe was nervous being there by himself, so toward the end one of us would stay with Joe and the other one go to the inn to sleep. Joe was in a semi private room with a man that had a heart transplant. We found out he was from our hometown of Norwalk, Ohio. He was having some trouble with leg swelling and had been there for a month.

The first day the interns came in to see Joe, they told us he might have a hematoma at the sight of the surgery and if they couldn't stop the bleeding, they would have to open him up in surgery and drain it out. A hematoma after surgery is usually the result of damage to the blood vessels during surgery or poor patient aftercare.

If the case is not severe, it usually clears up in several days. Otherwise, if the hematoma gets bigger, it cuts off the oxygen to the surrounding tissue causing necrosis or death to the vessels. This hematoma was right next to the new kidney. We were all upset by this but they said they would watch his red blood count and maybe it would go away by itself. We saw his surgeon for about five minutes while Joe was in the hospital and did not see him again at all.

The interns came in the next day and said they were going to give Joe a transfusion for the blood loss caused by the hematoma. By the end of the week, they said Joe's red blood count was alright. What we didn't know then was that of course the red blood count would read alright because of the transfusion, but that did not mean that the hematoma was gone. His kidney function tests were ok at the time and they said he could go home.

Joe was told to stay home and away from the public for a month after the transplant to prevent any exposure to sickness or infection. He also had a lot of pills he had to take three times a day. They put him on a new drug called Rappamune, which was an immunosuppressant drug for kidney rejection. A stent was also put in his urethra during the surgery to keep the tube open from the kidney to the bladder. This would be removed in a couple months. The surgeon had removed the peritoneal tube in his stomach in surgery, so all he had left was a JP drain in his side at the site of the surgery.

Three days after the surgery, Chris was still in pain. The pain pills were not working and she couldn't eat like she was supposed to. The male nurse on her floor said she was a big baby who couldn't stand pain. We didn't really know how bad the pain was. We all thought maybe it was because she had never had surgery before, and didn't know what to expect. After four days, she still couldn't eat, but sent her home anyway.

When Joe got home, we were so happy there was no more dialysis. Harry and I took the remaining dialysis bags out and smashed them in the backyard. It was like a celebration.

After a day or two, there seemed to be constant issues with him. The stent in this urethra was bothering him, and he looked so pale and weak. The site of the hematoma on his side was turning purple and red and getting bigger every day. Harry took a picture of it for evidence. We both thought that Joe should have looked a whole lot healthier by now, but he looked worse than when he was on dialysis.

During Joe's first post-op appointment with the surgeon, we pointed out the hematoma. The surgeon said it was just blood under the surface of the skin and it was normal. I realize now he must have known it was not normal for it to look like that after two weeks. And he let him go home that way.

When Chris got home, she felt awful. She noticed that her main incision where the kidney had been taken out was much lower than they had said it would be. And it seemed to be swollen as if it had a lump in it. Her abdomen was still so bloated from the air they put in her for laparoscopic surgery. She just felt so full, as if no food would fit in her stomach, and could not breathe when she lay down.

On her first post-op visit, her surgeon just said that everything was normal and that she still had air in her. He just ignored what she was saying about her incision, so she pulled down her pants and forced him to look at it. His eyes got big and he sent her down to x-ray where they extracted a sample of fluid out of her incision and found out she had a staph infection.

She went back up to the doctor's office again and he opened up a slit in her incision and showed her how to pack it with gauze. He then started writing a prescription for an antibiotic for the infection, and asked her if she was allergic to any kind of medication. Right away she said penicillin, and went home with the prescription, which Norma took to the drugstore.

They got a call an hour later from the pharmacy saying Chris could not take this medicine. The prescription was for very strong penicillin and it could kill her. Was the doctor not listening or was he trying to hurt her on purpose?

Chris was very upset because she would have no medicine until morning and she was afraid of the doctor and his motives. In the morning, she called the doctor's nurse and they called in a new prescription.

When Nancy and Norma went to their doctor's appointment and told them Joe also had kidney disease, he wanted our family to have genetic counseling because so many members of the family had kidney disease. Harry was against it, but we had Jon's kids, and our own future grandchildren to consider. Of course, they wanted our appointment filmed so they could publicize it.

Carol was not in favor of doing this either, but her and Jon came that day. I felt that Joe should not be out in public so soon, but we went into a side door and right into the doctor's office. We always felt like we were doing the right thing for our family. We were so messed up in the head over kidney disease; we always made the wrong decisions. Joe didn't feel too good earlier that day, but he went with us. He was starting to have pains in his arms and legs and felt weak.

The media guy filmed us going into the building and sitting in the waiting room. They filmed Jon's kids like they were the next generation of kidney patients. It just turned my stomach. The family all filled out questionnaires about their transplants and they all had urine and blood samples taken.

It was explained to us that scientists had narrowed down this disease to several different chromosomes. This disease has a fifty-fifty chance of showing up in the children of people with this disease. And if you are a family member that does not have the disease like Mike, you cannot pass it on. They asked us at the end if we had learned anything today, and Harry said yes, "If these are the odds, we are not very lucky."

The doctor wanted one member of the family to have a $2000.00 test done on one of their chromosomes to test for this disease, and they weren't even sure this would be the right chromosome. They wanted us to pay for it, and told us health insurance wouldn't cover it since it was experimental. None of us had that kind of money. We all thought that if the Cleveland Clinic wanted these kind of experiments done they should be paying for it.

What a crock of shit and a waste of our time was all we could think. They said they would take the results of the urine and blood samples and send them to other hospitals that were doing studies on kidney disease. We all went home shaking our heads in disgust; we just felt used.

Later on, everyone got a copy of the records we had filled out there, and the clinic had mixed them all up and mailed our copies to the wrong people. Jon had Harry's, and Nancy had Joe's, and so forth. What morons! They could not even get that right. It would be four years later before we ever heard anything about the studies they did and it told us nothing. Anyway, by that time we wanted nothing to do with the whole thing.

By now it was two weeks after

the transplant, Joe was getting sicker, his arms and legs had severe pains in them, and the purple bruise on his side was getting bigger yet. The clinic told us when Joe was discharged to tell them right away if Joe had any flu like symptoms. We called right away and the kidney coordinator said that so long as Joe didn't have a fever he was alright. Harry and I were worried. The next day he developed a fever, and we called right away. The male transplant coordinator there said Joe's two-week appointment was the next day so we could wait until then.

The morning of his doctor's appointment, Joe started to throw up and was really sick. He had to be taken in a wheelchair upstairs to his doctor's appointment. We told them how sick he was and still they let him sit out there and wait for two hours to see the doctor. We were beside ourselves by then. Joe had a terrible headache on top of everything else.

We finally got into the doctor's office and the intern saw how sick Joe was. He said he was going to suggest that Joe be admitted. When the surgeon came in and the intern told him about Joe, he just stood there and looked at him. The intern said, "well don't you think that he should be admitted?" The surgeon starting stuttering and said, "yeah, I guess so."

They made us go down to the lobby and wait until they found him a room. Joe was sitting in a wheelchair, sicker than a dog with a splitting headache. Joe's surgeon walked by a one point and looked at Joe, and said, "they'll find you a room," and walked on. He never even lifted a finger to help, even though he knew Joe was really, really sick.

Finally, two hours later, we badgered them enough that they found him a room on the bariatric floor. They said there were no rooms available on the transplant floor. They might as well have left him in the lobby. The nurses on that floor knew absolutely nothing about taking care of seriously ill people.

It took them an hour to bring Joe a pain pill for his headache. He was crying it hurt so badly. He was dehydrating from throwing up and we had to beg for an IV. He should have been put on the transplant floor where they would have hopefully realized the seriousness of his condition.

The next morning the interns came in and said they were going to run a barrage of tests to see what was wrong. It was suggested that the immunosuppressant drug Rappamune, that Joe was taking might be a problem, and that he should probably not be taking it. That night the nurse on the floor wanted to give Joe Rappamune again and I tried to stop her, but the doctors had left no orders, so she gave it to him anyway. No big surprise for the Cleveland Clinic. The doctors don't leave any orders, and the nurse is too lazy to call and find out if what we said could be true.

The next day they decided to call in the nephrologists because Joe's creatinine, the test to determine his kidney function, was getting higher. They came in and said they thought it could either be kidney rejection or the return of his kidney disease in the new kidney.

If I had one wish in that hospital, it would be for the interns to shut their mouths until they had a test to prove something. They are always throwing out random theories to the patients that scare them to death and are usually not true. When they were all done dishing out their bad news, they left to order the tests.

Another bad thing about being on the wrong floor was that the doctors would come and visit Joe last. The nurses on that floor also didn't realize that kidney patients had to have their pills at a certain time.

One day they were hours late giving Joe his pills. We just kept complaining, but they had to wait for the pills to come up from the pharmacy in the basement. They should have known when he was first admitted that he needed these pills every day.

One night they asked Joe for a urine sample. I took it down to the nurse's desk. It had a huge white cotton ball in it, which struck me really odd because I knew that it was albium. That's what leaks into your urine when you are in end stage renal disease.

The nephrologists came back in and said it had to be recurring kidney disease. Although we had been told that there is a small possibility this can happen, it would never have progressed as far as the urine sample suggested. We just discarded the whole idea as ridiculous; it had never come back in our family. They had no idea what was wrong.

Meanwhile, Chris was still at home bloated and sick. She made numerous calls to the Cleveland Clinic and got nowhere with her concerns. The doctor just kept prescribing pain pills without knowing why she was in pain. She finally went to her local doctor who ordered a cat scan for her.

The result was that she had what is called ascities chylous, which were lymphoecele leaks in her abdomen. She was full of fluid. They told her that she had to go back to the clinic because they created the situation she was in. She was very scared, she was afraid they would injure her worse than she already was.

Her surgeon at the clinic was forced to see her again. He told her this was nobody's fault, not hers and not his. Can you believe it? What an idiot! How could it possibly be her fault, and how could it not be his? As I understand it, this doctor has told many of the patients he has injured this same story. Only the guilty would suggest such a thing to his patients.

He sent her to x-ray to have an ultrasound-guided aspiration. In layman's terms, they stuck a needle the size of a crochet hook in her stomach to draw out the fluid. Chris said they had to hold her down because she couldn't breathe and it hurt so badly. She said she could feel the needle go through every layer of flesh. It just makes me sick. They removed 1800cc's of milky white fluid that first time.

She had to be aspirated every week and the fluid just kept filling back up inside her. On her last visit to this horrible monster, he told her he thought the fluid was subsiding and didn't need any more aspirations. He came to this conclusion by just looking at her, not by having any tests done. Chris knew better, she was still bloated and miserable. I guess this was his way of telling her he was washing his hands of the whole situation.

Meanwhile, the transplant surgeon on rounds came in and said he thought Joe needed a biopsy of his kidney to see what was going on. He kept pushing the theory of the return of kidney disease, and Harry had just about had enough of their bullshit and told him "get the out of here and don't come back."

If you could see these arrogant assholes, the picture you would get is of them strutting back and forth across the room spouting theories almost as if they were on a stage performing. The ironic part of this is that they have no clue whether they are right or wrong. They are so full of themselves that they never even notice what effect their words are having on the patient.

Joe had the biopsy and they said it showed rejection. We would later learn that this was also a lie. The real result was acute tubular necrosis, damage to the tubular cells of the kidney. So, they said they were going to give him thymoglobulin treatments that you use for rejection and assured us they can always turn this around.

After that, Joe was transferred to the transplant floor. The first night he was there, he had terrible pains in his arms and legs. He was just screaming and nothing they gave him numbed the pain. I could feel myself breaking out in a cold sweat. It was horrible to watch your child suffer this way and not know what is wrong with him. We had heard horrid stories from the night nurses that the drug Rappamune can cause this and that they had seen people carried away in the night from the side effects of this medicine.

After four hours of this, the pain subsided and no one offered any explanation as to why this had happened. The next day they decided to transfer Joe across the hall and he ended up in the room with the heart transplant patient from Norwalk again.

The following weeks are a blur of nightmares. A new nephrologist came to see Joe and we hated him. He was a smart-ass pretty boy with a huge ego. He brought in an infectious disease doctor who determined, but never really confirmed with a blood test that Joe had a blood disease called TTP. This is a disease that affects the antibodies and causes blood clots possibly blocking off blood flow to the kidney and making it fail. The nephrologist just kept telling us how sick Joe was and that this disease could be fatal. It was never proven one way or the other.

We didn't really believe that he had this disease either because the symptoms of kidney failure and this disease were similar. However, when they kept shoving the bad news in your face, it was hard to ignore. Joe was terrified. I could have strangled them with my bare hands; we were so mad, tired and scared.

I could not believe the same terrible nightmare was happening to Joe that had happened to Harry more than 30 years before. To be in the same hellhole and be told you were going to die. This should have never happened in this day and age. For Harry it was like reliving it all over again and he felt responsible.

How could Joe have gone from kidney failure to a deadly disease with no warning? Now we know that TTP was suggested to draw our minds away from what they really did. The symptoms were so similar that it was very convenient for them. That is sadistic and the product of very evil minds.

We stayed with Joe day and

night. We dozed in chairs if we could. There were just endless days and nights there, and I can remember every day the sun would come up over gloomy gray buildings. There never seemed to be any hope in sight.

The hospital rooms on the transplant floor were filthy. There was blood and urine on the floor. The curtains between the two beds had blood and filth on them. The nurses would drop the various needle and IV parts on the floor and they would just end up rolling under the beds and never be picked up.

There were not enough nurses to care for the patients, and the rooms were so small that there was barely enough room for the nurses to get next to the beds with all the equipment in there. And this is a transplant floor where everything is supposed to be so sterile. What a joke.

Then they decided to put Joe on plasmapherious, which cleans all the blood in your body and replaces it with fresh blood. They said this would help the blood disease. My poor child, the things they were doing to him. How in the world do you keep someone's spirits up in this situation? What can you possibly say to him to make anything better?

Joe had three thymoglobulin treatments, and the pills that they gave him after the last treatment had bad side effects. He started having delusions. He kept seeing people walking by in front of him when no one was there, and he didn't know where he was.

The same time this was going on his nose started bleeding profusely, I remembered the story of Harry's Uncle Herman, and his nosebleeds when they found out he had kidney failure. I remember it was late at night and we were sitting in the chairs outside of his room and he was talking nonsense and blood was running out of his nose, and we had to find some late night doctor to try and help him.

We finally found someone to come and look at Joe and he told us that the medicine was making him delusional and we would have to wait for it to wear off. Then he calls an ear, nose, and throat doctor to look at his nose. Then we had to wait for him to come. Of course, he had no clue why his nose could be bleeding. He gives him some drops and says to call him back if it doesn't work. They just kept covering up the ailment and never looked for the cause. By then, it was two a.m. It seemed every night was like that there. There was always a crisis of one sort or another going on.

We just kept asking to see the doctor that had operated on Joe, but he would not come to see him. The nurses were told to give Joe round the clock IV's to flush him with fluid to try to get the kidney to work. He was eventually so full of fluid that we had to cut his socks to fit them on his feet, and his testicles were the size of grapefruits.

One day they took a chest x-ray and we never knew the results. Joe's medical records would later tell us he had pulmonary edema, which meant his lungs were starting to fill up with fluid. They never told us what was really happening. They just kept spreading their lies so we didn't know what really bad shape Joe was in, and that it was their fault.

That's one of the really disgusting things there. When they have a deadly theory that is never based in any reality, they just love to run and tell you. However, when there is something really wrong and it is their fault, you never hear about it.

Then Harry spotted the idiot that operated on Joe in the hallway, and cornered him in the elevator. He told him "Joe is so full of fluid he can't breathe, don't you think he should be on dialysis?" The surgeon was nervous as hell and said, "Yeah, Yeah, I guess so." He knew Joe's lungs were starting to fill with fluid, and Harry had to tell him to do something.

Was he purposely trying to kill Joe? He was the one that filled him full of water, and then he doesn't want to do anything to help him. Total neglect and incompetence. How did he ever get to be the head of the department?

About this time, Chris called us from home and said she had gotten a copy of the movie of the surgery. The media department and transplant coordinator said we could have one. They were supposed to send us the edited version of the movie where the interviews we had given were intertwined with the surgery. Instead, the morons had sent the unedited version of the movie. All the better for us, thank God.

The surgeons had microphones on during the surgery and when the camera crew and people watching the surgery went on breaks, the camera and microphones were still on. Obviously, the doctors didn't know this because you could hear every word they were saying. Chris told us they had done a lot of things to injure her and the transplanted kidney. We were shocked, but it explained a lot about what was going on with Joe and Chris, we were on guard and very angry. We didn't tell Joe any of this at the time.

CHAPTER NINE

Shortly after that, Harry and I saw the head of nephrology when we were downstairs in the lobby. He had been Joe's doctor when he was on peritoneal dialysis. We asked him what in the world could be wrong with Joe; we had so many conflicting opinions. He said the kidney was injured, and we now knew why from what Chris had told us, but we asked him how this could have happened. We wanted to see what answer he would give us.

Of course, he never answered the question directly; they excel at avoiding the truth at the clinic. He just went on to explain that the kidney has thousands of nephrons that can be injured, and once they are injured, they never heal. It was now a question of how much function the kidney had left in order for it to work.

Well, we knew that was a bleak prospect and Joe would never be well with a half-functioning kidney. We knew those butchers had killed it during surgery somehow, but we had not seen the movie yet, and could not put the pieces together at the time.

So now, we had the infectious disease doctor continually coming in and telling Joe he had a blood disease and it was fatal, and the pretty boy nephrologist telling him that he was seriously ill. We didn't even know if any of this was true, but Joe was so sick and despondent. We tried to tell him we didn't think it was true, but how do you convince someone who feels so helpless? They just kept hammering at him every chance they got. He just kept hoping they could save his kidney, but by this time we pretty much knew that there was little hope of that.

Next, they came in and told him they were going to put a tube in his chest for hemodialysis. They took him downstairs to have it put in through a vein in his neck. Another surgical procedure, and it had three tubes coming out of it so blood could be taken from it also. His arm was so black and blue from blood tests and IV's that they were having a hard time getting any blood out of the veins anymore.

They brought him back up to his room and had to start using it right away, he needed dialysis so bad. They never plan ahead or consider the patient. If the tube had been put in sooner, it would have had some time to heal. Joe had his blood exchanged in the morning during plasmapheresis and had dialysis in the afternoon. They had to roll him in his bed to the treatments, because he was too weak and bloated to sit up in a wheelchair. What went on was just indescribable.

Then the tube is his neck kept bleeding. It was so bad we

had to sop it up with huge pieces of gauze and his bed was always full of blood. I changed his sheets four times a day. The nurses refused because they don't change beds after two p.m. You were lucky if they did it before that time; they were so slow. I guess if the patient is alone there, they just have to lie in filth until morning if their bed somehow gets dirty, and I imagine that happens quite often in a hospital.

Finally, we called an intern to come in and told him he had to do something about this bleeding. He came in and put these big huge stitches across the tube in his chest. He was still there when the doctor came in who had originally put the tube in. She asked the intern "what do you think you are doing? This is my patient, and someone should have paged me. You are putting the wrong kind of stitches in there."

He made some sort of feeble

explanation and then the two of them proceeded to shove each other and started screaming over the top of Joe's bed. We could not believe this was going on, we just stood there and looked at them. What would happen next in this hall of hell?

We had just about had it. I went down to the head nurse and complained about what was going on. They had a patient advocate on the floor to help the patients. Harry and I had a meeting with him and the head nurse and complained that no one in the place was on the same page. We had four or five different doctors and interns coming in, all with different opinions. Then we had these last two fighting over the top of Joe.

We demanded to see the surgeon who had operated on Joe. We wanted to know what was wrong with Joe and what they were going to do about it. We wanted them to talk together and come up with the same opinion and a plan, and have

one person from that point on to
take over Joe's care.

The next day we were told
that "the team" would come in and
talk to us. So, Joe's surgeon, two
interns, a transplant coordinator
and the pretty boy nephrologist
came in and gathered around Joe's
bed. My stomach was just turning
and Joe looked scared. His surgeon
said nothing; he just stared at
his shoes. Pretty boy was elected
to talk and he just spouted the
same old story. He just said Joe's
kidney was rejecting and he had a
blood disease and it just did not
look good.

They said they were going to
continue with hemodialysis and
plasmapheresis. They did not
reveal one bit of information
about why it was happening, but by
then we knew they had injured it
and were not going to admit it. We
never asked them one question, we
just looked at them. We knew then
that we were surrounded by the
enemy and they had closed ranks to

tell us a pack of lies. A wave of terror washed over me and I would have given anything to take Joe and get out of there. We were afraid for his life.

Not a half hour after that discussion of getting on the same page, the stupid infectious disease doctor came in and told Joe once again that he was dying of a blood disease. They obviously were not going to stop the horde of people coming in there. Harry told him to get out and not come back.

We had also asked the pretty boy nephrologist to please stop coming in and telling Joe he was going to die. He just would not stop; so much for patients rights in that hellhole. We asked to talk to the head of nephrology again, who was his boss, and asked that he please stop this asshole from harassing Joe every chance he got.

Our request was totally ignored. The asshole just waited until Joe was on dialysis and went in there to harass him instead. He knew we couldn't come in there, and Joe was too weak to argue with anyone. We hated that bastard.

Harry and I had been awake for weeks now and the stress was killing me. I started getting sick; I threw up and had diarrhea so bad that I couldn't stay there. This was during one of the times Chris was in Cleveland for more tests. Therefore, I went home with Nancy, Norma, and Chris. Chris gave me one of her phenergans, which is a stomach relaxer to take so I could make it home without being sick in the car. I never take anyone's medicine, but I just didn't care by this time.

I remember getting out of the car at home and I looked around. It was early May, and everything was blooming. The lilac bushes and all the flowers were just beautiful. I wondered how so much beauty could exist in the world of ugliness I had been living in. I just started to cry. I so badly wished we could all come home and live our normal lives there again.

I went into the house and everything was just the same as when we left, but it all just seemed unfamiliar. I didn't think I would ever look at anything the same here again. Between no sleep and the pill, I fell instantly asleep. My mother tried to call me and I didn't know who she was. I slept for fourteen hours straight. I knew it was stress because except for being extremely weak I was ok.

It took me five days to get back to Cleveland. Harry was there alone and so scared. We asked Mike to come and be with his dad. During this time, Joe's stool was jet black and no matter how many times Harry mentioned that no one seemed to care. Obviously, he was bleeding internally somewhere, probably from the hematoma. But no one was talking about that anymore; the subject was totally ignored, even though the hematoma was still there.

Once when Joe was being rolled down the hall to go to dialysis, his surgeon happened to be there. Joe asked him why this was happening to him, and the doctor said, "This is no place to talk about this," and just walked very quickly down the hall away from him. He absolutely refused to talk to him or discuss this subject at all, because he knew he was guilty as sin.

The interns said that they had never seen anything like what was happening to Joe. Of course not, who would dream that they had injured the kidney during surgery and put it in a person anyway. Joe had a renal scan to search for a urinary leak. There was a large pocket of fluid around the kidney, but no urinary leak. They tried to drain the fluid and there was so much in there that they couldn't get it all out.

Next, they did an angiogram of the renal artery that is

connected to the kidney. This is a scan to check for any blockages that might damage the kidney. Reading his medical records later, we found out the kidney was surrounded by so much fluid that his bladder was being shoved to the left and was causing uremia. This is a high level of waste or poison in your blood that leads to sepsis, which could have killed him.

The last test they did was a cat scan of his pelvis where they had put the kidney. The result, which of course we never heard about, was that there was no live tissue in the kidney, it appeared to be black; so in other words it was totally dead. There was more fluid than before; and it was in his peritoneal cavity, under his skin, and in the tissue anchoring the kidney to his stomach.

Joe asked Harry why God hated him. He said Joe was begging "Please Daddy, don't let me die, please don't let me die," and

271

asked Harry to lay his hand on his kidney so that it would be healed. Harry said he could see himself in the past when he had thought he was going to die. He was suffering all over again through his son. I should have been there. Joe was beyond miserable.

That murdering son of a bitch doctor had gotten that last report and did nothing. It was obvious that he wanted Joe to die to cover up his mistakes. He put him through all the torture he did so he could pretend that he was trying to save the kidney. He knew from the beginning it was dead and could have taken it out and saved him all that pain, torture and suffering.

The doctors were spreading the lie about the blood disease, so when Joe was gone they could use it for the phony cause of death. If that is what their so called "world class care", you can have it.

Chris meanwhile has realized

that her doctor is not going to do anything to help her. He wanted her to go on TPN, total parental nutrition, to heal herself. He told her she could go back to work then. Chris worked in a factory, and he wanted her to carry a feeding bag around with her while she worked. TPN was something that needed to be done under sterile conditions. Of course, consider the source; he didn't care about her or her life.

Nancy called me on my cell phone one morning and asked if we could find Chris another doctor to help her. I called one of the kidney coordinators and demanded that they find someone to help her. They made her an appointment with a vascular surgeon at the clinic. She really didn't want anything to do with any other doctor there, but we all knew that if she didn't have a clinic doctor fix her, they would say someone outside the clinic had injured her and not them. No one else in another hospital would touch her anyway.

Three days later another transplant surgeon came on rounds to see Joe. He also obviously saw the results of the CAT scan, but he wanted to do another biopsy. He did it in the hospital room. The piece he took of Joe's kidney was not big enough, so he had to do it again.

I can only guess he put him through the extra torture of a biopsy so he could pretend he had just discovered what was wrong and no one could blame him for what went on before. He said he would have the results in four hours and Joe went to dialysis.

Harry and I walked outside for the first time since we had been there. We needed to clear our heads and talk about what was going on. And wouldn't you know the first time we walked away, the doctor goes in dialysis and tells Joe the results of the biopsy. He tells him the kidney is dead and has to come out. Joe is crying when we get there. He cannot believe he has gone through all this for nothing. I will never ever forget the look of disbelief on his face. And I will never forget or forgive the clinic.

Chris was also heartbroken that nothing could be done to save her kidney, and she was also sick for no reason. We all dreaded telling her, and I didn't want to just tell her over the telephone. Nancy told her and Chris started to cry, and asked if nothing could be done to save it. She knew it was the clinic's fault and not Joe's. All her suffering was also for nothing.

When we got back to Joe's room, the interns tell us Joe should go home and recuperate before the surgery. The doctor who did the biopsy came back, and told us Joe will never live if he goes home; the kidney had to come out that night. By this point in time, we were just relieved that Joe would at least be alive and not be tortured anymore.

It was May 12, five weeks after the transplant and the surgery to remove the kidney was at 7:00 p.m. The doctor came out afterwards, said Joe was fine, and that he had drained out the hematoma. He said we deserved to know what happened to the kidney, and they would all talk about it.

Well, of course, we never heard a word about it. But we didn't need to be told. Joe and Chris' medical records and the movie of the surgery told it all. The report of this last surgery would say the kidney was black, dead, and swollen. It had to be removed carefully so it didn't fall apart inside Joe and cause sepsis.

After about a week Joe was finally well enough to go home. Hemodialysis treatments were set up for him in our local town. He had a JP drain in his side again from the last surgery to drain out any infection, a tube in his neck for dialysis and no kidney.

Their parting words to him were "Well you win some, you lose some." And that it would be much harder to get another kidney transplant now because he had some of Chris's antigens in his body. We wouldn't want to leave without one last zinger of bad news, now would we? They called the patient advocate on the floor to wheel Joe downstairs to the car. The nurses usually do this. I guess they wanted to see what we would say. We didn't give him a clue.

We pulled up in the driveway at home, and the first thing Joe saw was the swimming pool we had put in last fall. He would not be able to go in it because he had the dialysis

tube in his neck. That also meant none of us would go in the pool that summer. We couldn't go in there and leave Joe in the house alone. We had all waited years for a pool and that was just another thing the Cleveland Clinic took away from us that year.

Joe went in the house very angry and the first thing he saw was everything that he had been given for a present after his transplant. He threw everything away, went in his room, and slammed the door. We buried our own feelings so we could take care of Joe and deal with the mental state he was in.

We were finally at home and had a chance to really look at the movie of the surgery and we were shocked speechless. It was taped while a group from UNOS and some members of the Cleveland Clinic transplant team were observing. Chris and Joe's surgeons introduce themselves and say they have done over three hundred of these surgeries together.

Chris's surgeon takes over and points to Chris who has already been prepared for the removal of her kidney. Her surgeon is standing there bragging about his expertise in this field. He is stating that the recovery rate is much faster in laparoscopic surgery, how fast donors heal, how long they are off work and all kinds of statistics about kidney donors, none of which turn out to be true in Chris' case.

The surgeons move on to the removal of the kidney which they call" harvesting the kidney." That to me had a bad sound to it. Both of them are standing there, and Chris' surgeon has on short surgical gloves. Joe's surgeon says, "the ambiance in the room is that of a delivery." Chris's surgeon reaches inside of Chris with his hand instead of the silk bag he said he was going to use. Since her incision is a lot farther down than it was supposed to be, he had a long way to go to pull out that kidney. It is obvious that he squeezed too tight with his hand and injured the delicate nephrons of the kidney.

The kidney is put on a plate and Joe's surgeon says, "it's a girl" and holds up the kidney. Chris's surgeon is standing there with blood on the arm of his scrubs where he put his hand inside of her. Right there we saw the reason for the staph infection and lymphocele leaks. The rough material of his scrubs had scraped the inside of her. And this is supposed to be minimally invasive surgery!

Then Joe's surgeon takes over sitting at a table and preparing the kidney for transplanting into Joe. He had a microphone attached to him and the clinic employees were asking him questions. It was not a good idea in the first place to be answering questions during surgery and the stupidity of the questions being asked made it totally worthless. There should have been complete concentration on the part of the surgeon, but the show had to go on.

The observers took breaks every so often, so when they came back, everything the doctor had just done had to be explained. Joe was in surgery much longer than he should have been and this is not in the best interest of the patient or the kidney. The schedule printed for the day of the kidney symposium showed coffee breaks, donuts and box lunches. If this had been treated as a serious operation, the people would have kept their asses in there and the operation would not have taken as long as it did.

When these people were on break, Joe's surgeon didn't know his microphone was still on and the camera was still running. He makes several derogatory remarks about how this exposure sucks, and he was up all night and doesn't want to afterward. He is saying that these people are on break too long and if they don't get going onto the next step of the operation, they will never get out of there.

The two other interns that were on the surgical team with him were in training. One of them was putting in a suture incorrectly with a knot in it. That was wrong and had to be done over. The other one was falling asleep and not paying any attention at all. The surgeon asked him "could you would please participate and pay attention." To which he replied, "I have been up for days and I am tired. "He should have been dismissed, but you can't do that with a show to put on. The publicity was the only important thing, not the safety of the patient.

Therefore, the surgical director can't take the pressure of all the publicity and the interns are half-asleep, and as in every other part of the hospital no one knows what the other one is doing. Who are these people and why are they allowed to work there.

Then the surgeon realizes that no implant biopsy was done on Chris' kidney before it was taken out of her. This has to be done before the kidney is taken out of the donor to rule out the possibility of disease. His reply to this is "Christ, we missed it. Well that's the beauty of television, we can edit it out." So long as he could cover it up, he didn't care about whether or not it would hurt Joe. Later he would tell the observers that it was such a good kidney that they didn't need to do a biopsy. I guess he had x-ray eyes and could see right through it.

This is against the law, because when Chris first got the movie, Joe was still in the hospital. I asked one of the doctors if the biopsy had been taken on Chris' kidney because I wanted to know what he would say. He said that of course it was done, because it was against the law not to do it, so that was just another lie they told us.

Meanwhile, the kidney is constantly oozing blood and they

are trying to cauterize it. The surgeon remarks that "every needle hole is bleeding, and it's going on too long to be safe. It's just like kidney failure ooze and has been going on the whole time." They cannot stop the bleeding, hence the reason for the hematoma that he didn't fix while they were in there. He keeps asking his assistants if they think the kidney looks any better, and you can tell that they don't think it does.

Then they find a big piece of fat near the area of Joe's bladder, and the surgeon wants to know what the heck it is. He said, "Is this something else that we're going to regret? Yeah, we are going to regret it." The medical reports will later state that there was an area of fat and fluid in there that pushed Joe's bladder to the left.

When they go to connect the kidney to the bladder the vein is oozing and they are having a hard time accessing it. The surgeon then realized the sleeping intern had given him the wrong size suture. He says, "Well it will be my fault, it's always my fault." Evidently, he does a lot of things wrong. He does not even know what he is doing and you can't depend on sleeping assistants to know either. You can tell he is not happy with how this part of the surgery is going either. This movie was enough to give us nightmares for life.

Suddenly all the pieces were fitting together about what had happened to Joe. We were so angry we didn't know what to do with ourselves. We blamed ourselves first for taking Joe there. We felt totally betrayed by the people in those departments that we thought we had known for years and then turned their backs on us. They had used us for their own purposes and then threw us out in the trash just like they did Chris' kidney.

Joe had to go back to the clinic a week after he was home for his follow up appointment. We knew what that bastard doctor had done to him then, so we decided to bait him with questions. First, we asked him for a copy of the surgical report. He had an assistant in there with him and was very nervous about giving it to us. He said that maybe he could send it to us later on. His assistant just looked at him as if she was wondering what was wrong with him and said, "It could be copied off the computer right now. Why wait?"

Therefore, we had that in our hand, and then we asked him what we were supposed to tell people about what happened to Joe's first kidney, because no one had ever told us like they promised they would. And after all, we needed a new donor and people were going to ask us questions. He just looked at us, stuttered and stammered and said, "I'm going to have to look back over Joe's medical records and call you." As he forgot what had happened that whole last month to one of his patients. Call us indeed, we knew he would never put down anything in writing or call us.

We told him that it didn't help any that Chris' doctor had stuck his arm in her with his dirty rough scrubs. He just stared blankly at us, shook our hands, said "nice to meet you" and ran from the room. We just looked at each other, and said, "What the hell was that? Did he just meet us?" He must have ran from the room either to pull himself together or to call Chris' doctor. He looked guilty as hell.

His report for this appointment said Joe was still seeing the clinic doctors for his blood pressure issues, but he wasn't; they had washed their hands of him. Again, no one ever knows what the other one is doing there.

This was due in part to their

new electronic medical records, and what a mess that was. The various departments didn't know what the other one was doing already without these new records. The wrong tests and doctors notes and medications get put in the computer. The problem comes about in the translation from the person who is speaking and the person entering the information. This makes things even more screwed up than before.

When we got home we read Joe's surgical report, his doctor called what happened acute rejection, which means a mild one. It also states there were no significant findings in the first scan of the kidney. Not true! What about the fat plane turning the bladder sideways, the hematoma, the edema near the kidney transplant, the stranding and thickening of the urethra, and the fluid around the kidney? Then it states that he did everything he could, but the kidney failed anyway.

I would say he did plenty. He put an injured kidney in Joe and then tortured him unmercifully pretending to save a dead kidney and telling him he had a blood disease that was killing him. It was all a lie. Then it stated that there was no TTP. Finally, at the end, he admits there was no blood disease. The rest was a nice fairy tale, but as far from the truth as possible. They don't remove a rejected kidney and it doesn't turn black from acute kidney rejection.

How they ever thought they could get away with this I'll never know. They are liars and murderers and they have gone unpunished to do it to somebody else. And how many more people have they done this to? We would later find out and the numbers would be shocking.

A week later, the moron called us and said Joe's kidney failed because of rejection and TTP, the blood disease. He couldn't even remember his own lies. I said nothing, as I was the one on the phone. I didn't expect the truth, but I just wanted to see what the idiot would say. He just told me to keep looking for more donors.

CHAPTER TEN

Joe started on dialysis at the local center in town. In the beginning, Harry and I would sit in the waiting room and wait for him, and sometimes we would go in and sit with him when he was on dialysis to make sure he was alright. I think the nurses there thought we didn't trust them. In a way, they were right. They just didn't understand what we had all been through.

The nephrologist from the dialysis center came to see the patients every week, and checked their medications and their charts to see if the dialysis machine was cleaning the poisons out of their blood well enough. Then he would make some adjustments if they were necessary.

Joe was very angry that he had to be on dialysis there. Harry and I tried to explain Joe's anger to the nurses. It was not only the fact that he had kidney disease, but the loss of the transplanted kidney and all he had been put through at the Cleveland Clinic. The doctor put Joe on Paxil to help calm him down. It was just heartbreaking to watch. He would come home aching and tired, and he sometimes felt too sick to go back there again, but he had to. We had to bury our own emotions so that Joe wouldn't see how devastated we were. His morale was low enough.

Carol was at the dialysis center with Joe, and would watch out for him. Her kidney had failed a couple of years before that. Her son Jon had already had his transplant. I felt sorry for her; she had to sit there with her son on dialysis until he had his transplant, and now sit there with Joe. I myself could not have dealt with watching both of them.

The hardest part was keeping quiet about what we knew. We could not confront the clinic right away because we had information to find and we didn't want them to cover it up. Also, Joe still needed another kidney transplant, and you can't burn all your bridges. Harry was still a patient at the clinic, Joe still had two more follow up appointments, and Chris needed help.

Going to those final post-op appointments there was like going into enemy territory. You had to constantly watch your back, because we were in a nest of liars and killers.

Chris had been going to see the vascular surgeon and was told she would need additional surgery to repair the leaks and rips inside her. The doctor told her he was sick of fixing the mistakes the other doctors kept making. She had the surgery in June of 2006, and afterwards thought she was on the way to recovery.

The day after the surgery, the doctor who had injured her called her on the phone and told her she had to go on TPN. She told him that she thought this would not happen since she had the surgery. He just curtly told her she had to go on it to heal the inside of her. She was just crushed, one thing after another. She thought she was done with her original doctor. She felt used, betrayed, and had no respect left for him.

Chris went on TPN until the end of June. It was so hot and she could not eat or drink anything. She had to suck on ice to keep her mouth wet, but couldn't swallow it. Nancy was living with her at the time, and she had to go to other people's houses to eat, so Chris wouldn't see her. I could sympathize with that, we had done the same thing when Harry was on TPN.

After that, Chris started to feel worthless, like she didn't do a good thing after all. She had suffered through all that pain and misery and her kidney was dead. She hadn't helped Joe, she was still off work, and her life was bad. What was supposed to be a happy summer with everyone well, turned out to be one full of anger and disbelief over what had happened. None of us could have made it through this if we hadn't known what had really happened to them. The clinic had gotten away with too many things in the past, but this time we had the proof.

Chris and Joe said next to nothing to each other. Both of them were on antidepressants and did not want to talk to anybody. I called every day to see how Chris was, and she refused to come to the phone. Joe didn't want to talk to anybody either because we all just kept talking about what had happened. After awhile, Chris took offense to Joe not wanting to see anybody. It was nothing personal, and she actually felt the same way.

At Chris's last appointment with the vascular surgeon, she was taken off TPN and told she was finally healed. The doctor also told her that there was a chance that the mesh they put inside her to repair the leaks could tear again and for that reason she would never be able to carry a child. That was the last crushing blow. I guess the slogan of the kidney department at the clinic should be "donate life and we will take the life of your unborn children."

After that, Chris was finally able to go back to work. She had been off work four months, instead of the two months the clinic had told her donors usually take to be healed. She lost money, her self-esteem, and her kidney.

Chris naturally wanted to sue the Cleveland Clinic. All of the lawyers she consulted with said that she had one hell of a case and they felt so sorry for her, but they would not go against the

Cleveland Clinic. They stated that they could not disclose why. We could do nothing to help her because Joe had to have another kidney transplant and we didn't want to make any trouble right then. Chris was very upset and frustrated with this and we couldn't blame her.

We began to see more of the corrupt side of the system. Hospitals like this one are big business, and their business is keeping people from healing as long as they can so they keep coming back. And then of course, the lawyers are out to make money, and if they can make more money by letting the hospitals pay them off, they will. Most of them are on the side of whomever they can get the most money from.

Joe remained on dialysis through the summer. One of his friends was approved to be his donor and the surgery was to take place in November of that year.

During that summer, I had two

calls from the Cleveland Clinic. One was from the media guy who had filmed us having genetic research. He wanted to come to our house and film Joe for a final interview. I said absolutely not. He kept pressuring me to finish what we had started. He asked if we didn't want to know the results of the research. I said that we hadn't heard a word about it and probably never would. He finally gave up when I told him Joe's kidney had been killed and we wanted nothing more to do with them.

The second call came from the original person we had met with in the media department. They wanted our family to agree to a short program for the learning channel about a family with kidney disease. They wanted to come and stay at each of our houses for a couple of days to see life as a kidney patient.

Then they would go to the dialysis center and film Joe and Carol while they were on the kidney machine. Did they think that it was a fun time to come home every other day sick and tired and aching? Or to watch someone drink three very tiny cups of water a day and eat special foods? I just wanted to scream. Can you believe the absolute audacity of asking this? After that, they left us alone.

In September, the dialysis tube in Joe's neck was going bad. It had been placed in the carotid artery in his neck. They can only be used for so many months, but we were hoping it would last until the next transplant. But it had to be taken out, and the doctor in town decided to put a temporary one in the other side of his chest that would last another month until the transplant.

The tube that the clinic had put in was taken out and we were told to change the dressing the next day. The next morning just happened to be Joe's twenty-third birthday. Harry went to change the dressing and was shocked to see that the wound was so large. There is usually a small slit in the artery. We could see now see why that tube kept bleeding and needed extra stitches in it after it was put in at the Cleveland Clinic. We should have never been asked to change this bandage.

The minute the gauze came out, blood starting shooting out of his neck. The back of the couch was covered in blood. Harry yelled to call 911. The rescue squad came and took Joe, and Harry and I followed in our car behind. I happened to look across the street at one point and saw Mike going in to work. I was so happy that he knew nothing about what was going on, although later he would tell me that he had a bad feeling that something was wrong that day.

When we got to the hospital in our hometown, they rushed Joe in and started working on stopping the bleeding. Since the wound was so large, they were having a hard time getting the blood to clot. I was just hysterical and sick to my stomach. I thought Joe was going to die on his birthday.

Finally, the vascular surgeon came and got the bleeding to stop. They took him to a room for a couple of hours to make sure he was ok. They offered him some birthday cake to try and cheer him up, but he was mad that he had to be there at all, much less on his birthday. He didn't want any cake and started yelling about what he called "the Greiner curse," which was kidney disease, and why did he have to have it.

Shortly after that, his second transplant was scheduled. We were not going to let either of the original surgeons within ten feet of Joe and the new donor. It was too late to start over in another hospital. A week before the surgery, Joe and his friend had the final blood tests to make sure their blood was still compatible.

The original surgeon called and said the blood tests did not look good; his friend was no longer a match. How were we going to tell Joe this latest bit of bad news? He was really heartbroken and depressed. The pre transplant coordinator from the clinic that Joe had seen told us that they were surprised; the match was still a good one. So what was this doctor up to now? Obviously, he didn't want Joe back there again.

During this time, Chris came over and said she had found a lawyer and a tentative court case was scheduled. We had wanted her to wait until we could present a combined case together that would explain her injury and the reason the kidney had died inside Joe. Time was running out for Chris to sue the clinic for malpractice as you only have so much time to do this after you are injured. And we understood this.

As it turned out anyway, the lawyer called her and said he was dropping the lawsuit. She asked him why and he wouldn't tell her. There are local lawyers that sit on the board at the Cleveland Clinic and it is very hard to sue the clinic with a lawyer from Cleveland. And her lawyer had let the statue of limitations run out on her case and it was too late to sue them.

In the winter of 2007, the tube in Joe's neck was about used up and had an infection in it. He was admitted to the hospital in our town and put in ICU. Someone had to come from Mansfield, which is a nearby town where the kidney doctors were located and put him on dialysis while he was there.

The dialysis nurse thought that maybe his gallbladder was acting up; she said that sometimes happens when there has been a lot of trauma to the body. Harry and I sure hoped not, Joe did not need to have any more surgery at the time. It turned out to be alright and I wondered then if that was why Harry's gallbladder had gone bad so soon after his aneurysm.

It was time for Joe to have a fistula for dialysis put in his arm. Joe did not want this done because it seemed so permanent. But there were no more donors left; the clinic had scared off the rest of them by not answering their phone when they were trying to offer a kidney. Some of them were wary because of what had happened to Joe. Everyone in town knew by now because Chris was injured.

Well hindsight they say is twenty-twenty. If we had known Joe would end up being on dialysis for nearly two years, we would have agreed to have a fistula put in when it was first brought up at our local hospital when Joe was first diagnosed with kidney disease. Now it had to be done anyway. All those tubes he had put in his body for nothing. An appointment was made with a vascular surgeon in our town for the procedure.

Joe had the fistula put in his arm shortly after that. The vein wasn't big enough and he had to have it done again. Then, of course, he had pain in his arm because it had to be used right away. There was no time to let it heal at all. That caused a few rough dialysis treatments.

This was a most heartbreaking time for all of us. The sadness and disillusionment we felt were almost overwhelming. We had to stay positive for Joe and hide our own emotions. This caused Joe to be angry sometimes, because we tried to stay cheerful and it seemed like we did not understand what he was going through. But it wouldn't have been good for him to see how devastated we were. At one point, we wished we could just kill ourselves, but we still had our kids to think of.

After that, things seemed to calm down and went along as they were supposed to. We started to look into putting Joe on the list at other transplant centers. We wanted to put Joe on as many lists as possible. We went to UTMC in Toledo and really liked the people there. Everything was organized, and Joe had all the tests done and was put on their transplant list, which had a lot shorter wait time than in Cleveland.

We transferred all of Joe's waiting time from the list in Cleveland to Toledo. Most of the hospitals in Cleveland were on the same list and it could have been a wait of three to five years. Toledo's list at the time was about eighteen months.

We waited through the summer comforting Joe the best we could. He could swim in the pool now since he didn't have a tube in his neck. That helped pass the time. They said that swimming helps dialysis patients feel like they have water in their body since they can drink so little.

Around this time, we starting

306

watching Joel Osteen. He really changed our view since our faith in anything was in really short supply at that time. Someone at work also gave Harry a copy of "The Secret" on DVD. Between those two things, we started to believe that Joe would get another kidney and he would be alright.

Harry kept believing that Joe would get a male kidney that was from someone his own age with a creatinine of 1.2 so that it would last a really long time.

Harry and I carried phones around with us everywhere waiting for the call for a kidney. On November 16, Joe came home and told us the Cleveland Clinic had called him and said they had a possible kidney for him. He told them he would have to talk to his parents about it. We were just dumbfounded because we were planning on getting a call from Toledo. We didn't want to go back to the clinic. We had transferred all his time to Toledo and still he got a call from the clinic.

I called the kidney coordinator in Cleveland and asked for details. She said a man of 28 had died in Florida and the kidney was a zero mismatch for Joe. Which meant it was identical to his own kidneys, which comes around once in a blue moon. There were only two other people in the United States that it matched.

One person who needed a kidney transplant and another one who needed a kidney and pancreas transplant. The other person who needed only the kidney would be called first. She would let us know. The surgeon that would do the surgery was the same one who had taken the dead kidney out of Joe before. I asked if they were positive this surgeon would do it and she said yes.

So the three of us sat down to talk about it. The donor, his age, and his creatinine level were identical to what Harry had believed Joe would get. It was a zero antigen mismatch, and the surgeon who had taken the dead kidney out would know how he had left things inside of Joe's body in preparation for another transplant.

But the Cleveland Clinic? That was a tough one. But our son was sick and suffering, and we didn't have much of a choice. Especially when they called back and said one of the people had said no, and the kidney matched no one except Joe.

We were told to be in Cleveland the next morning for the tests Joe needed prior to having a transplant. By late afternoon, they said everything was fine with Joe and they were just waiting for the kidney to come in from Florida. I assumed the young man had died at the Cleveland Clinic in Florida and that is why only they had the kidney.

Joe was so nervous because of where he was. He was so afraid they would hurt him again and then

he would die. He had to be
sedated. My feelings were so
mixed, but I did not feel the
dread that I felt the first time.
We waited and waited and finally
the surgery started at 11:30 p.m.
on November 17, 2007.

Harry and I got to wait in a
small room outside the OR this
time because the surgery center
waiting room was closed for the
night. Thank God, I hated that
room, and it was a lot calmer
sitting in that little room. And
this time we were not waiting for
the results of two people in
surgery.

In a couple of hours, the
surgeon came out and said that Joe
was fine and everything had gone
well. The kidney was in his left
side this time. He was back in his
room by that afternoon. Joe had to
be given thymoglobulin treatments
again. They do that with a cadaver
kidney to give it a jump-start
because it has been out of the
body of the original person for a

day before it is transplanted. After a couple of days, we went home.

We were not home twenty-four hours when Joe started to feel achy. The pain kept getting worse in his arms and legs, and we just thought, here we go again. We took him right back to Cleveland to the ER; we didn't call ahead or wait for anyone else's opinion. We got there in the afternoon and the pain had gotten worse since we left the house.

They kept giving him pain pills and nothing worked. The transplant surgeon on rounds gave up their rule of never coming down to the ER and came with his interns. I thought that was very strange at the time, but dismissed it from my mind as there were more important things going on.

They said he had serum sickness from the thymoglobulin. He had a reaction to it because it was still in his system from the year before. Harry and I just thought that if they hadn't given it to him for a dead kidney this would never be happening now. They said it would take two to three days to pass, but he would be alright.

The rest of that day was a nightmare of pain for Joe. By the time he got to a regular room the nurses were ready to change shifts, so no one was going to do anything for him until the night nurses came on. When they finally did, his nurse just kept telling him she could not give him any more pain medicine, she had given him the limit.

She said the pain management team would have to come in and there was only one group of them in the hospital, and he would have to wait his turn. Only one pain management team in the entire clinic? Wouldn't you think that should be a priority? That sure tells you that they don't care if you are in pain or not. Joe was begging us to help him. I kept talking to him so he would focus on me and not the pain. It didn't work.

The head nurse on the floor at night came in with her bad attitude and told Joe there was nothing she could do for him until the pain people came. Joe was complaining and who wouldn't be at that point. That fat nurse looked at Joe and told him "You had just better just change your attitude." We just looked at her and Harry said, "You had better change yours if you want to keep your job."

Morning came and I went straight to the ombudsman's office to demand that the pain people come and see Joe. They usually have no choice but to listen to you if you have a patient in the hospital. Once you are out of there, they could care less what happened to you. Harry meanwhile was in Joe's room and told one of the doctors "If you don't get those pain people here right now, I'll own this fucking hospital!"

The pain people were there before I could even get back to his room. Joe was on such a high dose of pain medicine he was totally out of it. But at least he was not crying in pain anymore and that was all that mattered.

Because of the pain Joe was in, his creatinine level climbed up a couple of points. The nephrologists came and thought this was to be expected due to the pain he was in. However, as before, the surgeons were on a different page. They wanted to do a biopsy on his new kidney. Harry and I were totally against it. Harry told the doctor "if anything happens to Joe I am going to own this hospital."

Instead of taking Joe down to the basement where they usually do these procedures, they took him upstairs to the procedure room in the outpatient nephrology offices. We thought at the time that this was very odd. The whole transplant team was in there to prep him for the procedure. It was then we realized they were scared of something. Obviously, they all knew what had happened before and were being very, very careful with him.

We realized then that they probably knew about Chris trying to sue them, so that is really why they were scared. Their concern wasn't for Joe at all, but for themselves. We had always secretly thought that if Chris proceeded with a lawsuit they would take it out on Joe, but evidently it helped him.

I was very upset during this biopsy and Harry told me not to show Joe my fear. He was right, but I could not stand any more of this crap. They wanted Joe to sign a paper to be part of a study where they did a biopsy twice a year for statistics on the health of a new kidney transplant. We said no, we thought they must be out of their minds. But to them people are just guinea pigs anyway. The results of the biopsy came back fine, so it had all been unnecessary.

When I had been in the ombudsman's office, I had also complained about that nasty head nurse. When she heard about this, she sent the nurse assigned to Joe to come in and tell us that we would not be allowed to stay in Joe's room all night. We told her we were not leaving and to tell her she would be in more trouble than she was already in if she made us leave.

By then it was the end of November and we spent Thanksgiving Day in the hospital. The serum sickness was passing, and Joe was being weaned off the pain medicine. It was finally time for him to go home and be well.

After that, Joe had several follow up appointments with the transplant surgeon. They clearly knew nothing about the working of the kidney itself once it is transplanted. Some people at the clinic continue to see the surgeons instead of the nephrologists, for their follow up care.

So here, once again, the surgeons and the nephrologists are continually at odds and in competition with one another. There is just no code of proper post transplant care. There is no plan on what to do with the patients once they have their transplants.

After two months, it was time to get out of there. We told them that we were moving to Toledo and would be seen at the UTMC transplant center from then on. We still said nothing about what we knew. We wanted them to give us Joe's medical records with no arguments. Once we got them, we were at last done with the place.

We went downstairs to sign papers for Harry's medical records and left the building knowing we were done with them forever. It was the best feeling I had in decades. I hated that place from the first day I saw it. Finally, to be free of the place I had hated and wished to never see again!

CHAPTER ELEVEN

We then made an appointment for Joe in Toledo and had his medical records sent immediately. He was our first concern. We then paid $100.00 to have the rest of Joe's records sent to us. Harry was waiting for his medical records to be sent to Toledo. The transplant clinic in Toledo requested them also. The Cleveland Clinic kept saying they had sent a synopsis of them.

Obviously, thirty-five years of records could not be sent and we could not afford to pay for them. Harry's records just never came. Joe's on the other Hand came in the mail with a bill for $100.00.

I called Harry's doctor in Cleveland. I told his secretary

that Harry was not coming back there and that we wanted his medical records. She told me "hire a lawyer, that's what everyone else has to do." Well, just great, but not unexpected.

Harry had some papers with blood work and a summary of his past appointments, and we sent them to Toledo, and they accepted them, so that Harry could be seen by a doctor there. Even they could not believe that a hospital would not send patients medical records when they were requested by another hospital.

It was like a totally different world there in Toledo. Everyone was so nice, and they knew you by name and not by a clinic number. The doctors took time to talk to you and were not mandated by a certain time period they were allowed to spend with their patients.

There is a kidney transplant coordinator there that is on call twenty-four hours a day. It doesn't matter how long you have had your transplant, they are there to help you. You can always talk to someone if you have a problem and your new prescriptions are always called in on time.

Now that Joe was well and he and Harry were out of the halls of hell, we had to decide what to do about what the clinic did to Joe. I think one of the worst things was that we promised Joe that he would not have to suffer like Harry did during his transplant. They made liars out of us in our son's eyes.

And we felt guilty for ever taking him to that horrible place. In fact, we will feel guilty until the day we die. It should have been a good memory and a day to rejoice. Nearly eighty years after Harry's grandmother died of kidney disease, they took what was supposed to be a miracle and turned it into the same ugly nightmare. And it should never have been that way in this day and age.

One good thing that came out of all this is that I have changed how I feel about people with kidney transplants. When I married Harry, I didn't know him before his transplant. I didn't realize that some of Harry's traits are just the way he has always been.

I thought that all his precise carefulness was due his having a transplant. But I knew Joe before he had his kidney transplant, and he is the same as he always was. So now it doesn't seem like a science experiment anymore. This really opened up my eyes, and I guess I finally grew up.

We were so thankful that Joe was well. He told us that he hadn't felt this good in years. Nevertheless, we all felt like we had been through a war and had posttraumatic stress syndrome. We had all been through so much horror and near death experiences, not once but three times in that place. And all due to their incompetence. We will never be the same again. Our trust has been ruined. We find it very difficult to trust anyone now.

If anyone has ever had a sick child or been in our place, you will understand what we are saying. The way you look at the world is totally different after what we have been through. No human being should ever have the power to manipulate someone else's life or death. Evidently, the Cleveland Clinic has the audacity to think they have that power and are untouchable. The only power they have is to trick and deceive people. I think that access to the internet is changing all that.

By January of 2008, we were totally done with the Cleveland Clinic. What a glorious day! Some people reading this will probably think we asked for all our troubles by going back to the clinic so many times. But when a large institution puts so much money into advertising to try and convince the public that they are the best in health care, it's easy to be deceived.

In looking back, we now realize what a mistake we made in ever going back there, but at those moments in time, it didn't appear the same way. So we admit we were stupid, and our son suffered because we were foolish enough to take him there. Please, please don't make the same mistake with your loved ones.

When we received Joe's medical records and I started to analyze them for evidence of what had happened to Joe, I was totally appalled at what I saw. As I read the results of the tests they had taken on Joe, I knew for sure that they had told us a pack of lies. They had tortured Joe pretending to save a kidney that they knew from the beginning was dying.

I spent the next six months going over records and reading medical information so that I could come up with a report of exactly what happened to Joe. This may sound crazy to some people, but I believe divine intervention helped me to understand all that medical terminology. Call it whatever you want, but I know I could never have understood all that information without help.

It just poured into my head, and I would sit there at times speechless, seeing what they had done to him and how they thought they were so clever in the way they had mislead us. First, the unedited copy of the surgery of the movie had been given to us, and now all this information to understand what they had actually done. We considered it a miracle and something that we were meant to know. We later had all this information verified by doctors.

By June of that year, we had a written report of what had happened to Joe and Chris and we decided to confront the clinic with it. Harry, Mike and I went to

Cleveland and asked to speak to the CEO. We were referred to the Ombudsman's office and strangely enough, the person we met with was the patient advocate that had been on the hospital floor when Joe had his first transplant. He was now an Ombudsman. He had been one of the people we had complained to at the time.

We talked to him and an assistant for awhile, and gave them a copy of the report. He said he would investigate this matter with the doctors and the people involved and get back to us. He said he didn't know how long it would take. The next day he called us and wanted a copy of the movie. They could not even find one.

We waited almost three months before we heard from them again. They were supposedly investigating what went wrong, but really, they were looking for someone to blame and a way to get out of it. When the ombudsman called us back, he told us we would all be meeting with the clinic's top attorney.

Only Harry and I went that day. It was a woman attorney and the first thing she said to us was "Where is your attorney? Didn't they come with you?" We told her we didn't need one. She was not too happy. She had our report in her hand, and she assumed that we had this report made up by a doctor. Harry told her that I had written it. To that, she made no comment.

She looked at our report and remarked that although she was not a doctor, it appeared that they had done everything they could to stop the kidney from rejecting. We interrupted and told her it was not a rejection, to which she replied, "whatever." Then we discussed the surgery movie and she told us that hopefully other people might not see it the same way we did. It was all a bunch of double talk as the evidence was there.

She told us that we looked

like very angry people and she offered to let us talk to a psychiatrist at the clinic. Yeah, right, let someone there tell us we're crazy and none of this happened the way we knew it did. We refused and then she said maybe they could get someone from another hospital to talk to us. To even suggest that she would have to think that we were pretty stupid. They would probably put a phony nametag on a clinic doctor and say he was from somewhere else. We just told her, "we don't need anyone else to tell us more lies."

We asked her what they were going to do about these doctors and what they did to Joe and Chris. She replied, "We have thousands of workers here and we can't keep tract of everything that goes on." Then she pointed her finger in Harry's face and said, "This isn't the first time this has happened and it won't be the last, you just happened to be someone who found out the truth."

So in other words, just live with it. So sad, too bad.

Well we told her we were going to write a book about it so that no one else would ever be injured this way. She said if we did that, it would be detrimental to the Clinic. Like we would care. When Chris's case was mentioned she very smugly said, "Oh yes, I know of your sister's case." Just as if to say that she took care of that one. I have to wonder what kind of conversation she had with Chris's lawyer.

She was getting snippier as the conversation went on. She could not convince us to be calm and forget about the whole thing. Harry told her, "I might not be able to shut down this place, but I'll put a big wedge in the door before I'm done." The hell with her and the clinic.

It was bad enough that our family had to go through the emotional turmoil of another member having kidney disease, but then Chris who never had the disease lost one of her kidneys also. After all they went through; they were simply thrown to the side. They just closed ranks at the clinic to protect themselves.

Now that we are out of that hellhole, the clinic still to this day sends us pamphlets about kidney transplants and envelopes asking for money to support the hospital. Their motivation is always concerning money, not the patients. It's like a factory, or a big business there where they herd more patients through than they can possibly handle. It's no wonder insurance premiums have gone up so high. They bleed everyone who has insurance by having to do second operations and unnecessary procedures and tests.

You might say to yourself that all hospitals make some mistakes. It is probably true, but the clinics "so called" mistakes are blunders. They are totally unwarranted, foolish, and happen because of the arrogant, self-righteous way that the doctors train their students there. They never fix their blunders; they hide them or bury them. We have proven that with our surgery video.

The first thing we did after that was to contact UNOS, the united network for organ sharing. Their mission is to oversee organ transplants, to offer help to organ donors and their families, and, if needed, to educate transplant professionals. They said that at the time Chris donated her kidney, they didn't have services to help living donors. They felt sorry for her, but there was nothing they could do to help her. They were however, surprised at the things they saw in the surgery movie that we sent them. That was the end of that.

Next, I complained to KEPRO who are a peer review organization that protects the rights of Medicare patients because they had paid for most of Joe's medical bills. I was told they are not an organization that could bring any kind of disciplinary action against doctors and hospitals. They are there to educate them on better methods for patient care. They said they would investigate the matter, but the doctors had the right to disclose the information from us.

The result of the investigation was that the standard of care was not met in the case of Chris and Joe. But, of course, the doctors refused to let us know the results; they have to protect their reputations. I asked someone at Kepro how this could be fair, since we had initiated the complaint. Why is the doctor protected and not the patients? They told me it's wasn't right, but that is the way it is right now.

Next, we wrote to Medical Mutual, which at the time was Joe's secondary insurance and they would do nothing. I could only assume it was due to the fact that the clinic is one of their major customers and they don't want to lose money. Next, we contacted the Joint Commission, who is supposed to oversee hospitals in regard to patient safety and care, and the answer was that they could see nothing wrong.

The state medical board even protects the doctors. Most doctor's credentials and reports of any bad surgeries they have done are hidden from the public. The clinic and some of its doctors are voted number one in medical journals year after year. The truth behind that is that the clinic finds out what medical procedures are being voted on that year and the doctors in those departments vote on each other to be nominated. How can they lose? And naïve people believe this propaganda. It is just malicious, contemptible, fraud.

There is absolutely no one

out there who is willing to protect patient's rights. Certainly not any of the so-called organizations that are supposed to help you when something goes wrong in a hospital. Certainly no lawyers, no newspaper reporters.

The Cleveland Clinic board members consist of local lawyers, businessmen, and Cleveland news-paper editors, and Cleveland Clinic doctors. They have that covered, no help there. It is all just a waste of time, everyone seems to be under the influence of the Cleveland Clinic in one way or another. They can literally get away with murder and go unpunished. There is no justice in the medical systems, only corruption.

The news people and radio stations won't talk to you because the Cleveland clinic pays them big money for advertising and they don't want to lose their business. The newspapers in Cleveland are the worst. They won't even allow you the freedom of speech to post a blog about the Cleveland Clinic on their articles. The comments are removed immediately. This is like communism and totally unfair to our rights as citizens. The journalists in Cleveland have lost their integrity and are merely puppets as far as being told what can be printed in the newspapers.

We then starting thinking about how we could get the word out quickly about what had happened to us, and to keep it from happening to anyone else. We decided we would create a website. We did some research and came up with a good web company. Mike set it up for us, and Joe picked out the name. He aptly decided to call it Kidneytransplantkiller.com.

I then began to type in all the information and it was ready to be published on the internet by January of 2009. I divided it into parts, what happened to Chris, Joe and Harry. We also made videos in which Harry and I talked about what happened at the clinic. We asked Chris and Joe if they would also make videos of what happened to them. We put these and pertinent parts of the transplant surgery on the website.

There was an overwhelming response to this. People from all over the country who had been injured at the clinic came forward to talk about their injuries. These stories broke my heart. I cannot forget the stories, or the people they have happened to. The suffering and the anguish and loss of quality of life and loved ones. There is death, amputations, loss of organs, disability, badly botched prostate surgeries, and it goes on and on. There have even been doctors from other countries wanting to use these videos to show how not to do transplant surgery.

Some of the identical things that happened to us have happened to other people. Issues with the ICU, surgeons, the blood lab, the incompetent billing department, the hours sitting in a wheelchair down in radiology, the interns running around giving their inexperienced opinions, the uncaring nurses.

The only people that receive "world class care" are the celebrities and dignitaries from other countries. The clinic wants these people to advertise for them, and hopefully donate large sums of money to the clinic in appreciation. They are catered to because of their money.

Our website has become global. We have people from other countries reading it. We also have a lot of people in many different states with the name of our website on bumper stickers on the backs of their cars. We have business cards that are being handed out everywhere by those who have been injured in one way or another by the clinic. We do not want this to happen to any more people out there. And believe me;

we have driven an untold number away from that place.

If the Cleveland Clinic doesn't care about their kidney transplants anymore, then they deserve not to do any. The new transplant department there is in a small corner of the fancy new heart center. They have put transplants on the back burner in favor of their new "so-called" heart and vascular procedures. The paintings on the walls in there are worth a fortune. However, they claim to be non-profit. The CEO there makes a salary of untold millions each year.

Since 2008, Hilda has been in a nursing home. She had so many strokes that she couldn't walk anymore. She needed a lot more care. I'm not sure if she really understood about Chris and Joe because at the time she rarely spoke anymore.

In January of 2009, she was diagnosed with cancer of the liver. I think she must have known it, because after that she just gave up. On January 18, the whole family was there and she died. At last, she was free of her mental anguish.

In the summer of 2010, Carol had her second kidney transplant and it has been successful for her. It has been three and a half years since Joe's second transplant and he is also well. Our health is the most valuable thing in the world to us. It is more precious than gold.

Since Joe's transplant, we have talked to many people in the same situation. I don't like the subject to be the main focus of my life, but I'm not afraid of it anymore. It has already happened, and although I realize that it could again, I don't spend much time thinking that way.

Joe lost his job after the last transplant. He and Chris remain unemployed due to the bad job situation in our economy. Joe has applied for help with the BVR, which is the Bureau of Vocational Rehabilitation for assistance. The economy has even affected help for the disabled. However, hopefully they are better equipped to help people than they were when Harry went to the BVR facility as a teenager.

None of us are the same anymore. We still try to be kind and have some compassion for people. But in spending all these years spreading the word, we have kept this issue alive. And we will be doing so forever.

We have tried to move on, but we never will totally. You really can't when there was no closure, no apologies, no compensation, nothing. The apologies would not have been sincere anyway. I have heard the same thing from many, many other people who are fighting their own medical battles with the Cleveland Clinic.

Joe and Chris find it very difficult to speak of it at all. Joe still has some nightmares about what the clinic did to him. Chris does not speak to us at all. Someone told us that when transplants within a family go bad, it tears the family apart. This went bad because of the Cleveland Clinic, but it still has the same effect.

It is now January 26, 2012 and Harry has had his kidney transplant for forty years. They have written an article about him in the local newspaper. I am proud of him for this accomplishment. He has taken good care of himself and this is a day to celebrate. I wish I could have foreseen this day when we were first married. But in the end, my wish for him came true anyway, and this day is the proof of it.

www.ingramcontent.com/pod-product-compliance
Lightning Source LLC
Chambersburg PA
CBHW060541200326
41521CB00007B/441